FULL LIFE

A WORKBOOK FOR SPIRITUAL RECOVERY FROM ADDICTIONS

by Francis A. Martin, Ph.D.

Green Hills Press
Nashville, Tennessee
www.greenhillspress.com
© 2010 Dr. Francis A. Martin

Cataloging-In-Publication Data
Martin, Dr. Francis A.
Full Life: A Workbook for Spiritual Recovery from Addictions
ISBN: 978-0-9661317-9-6
1. Non-Fiction 2. Self Help 3. Addiction 4. Religious

Published with the services of Grave Distractions Publications:www.gravedistractions.com
Cover, Interior Layout, and eBook conversion:
Brian Kannard

Editorial Note: Substance abuse is a serious illness that may require medical or other professional services. The author urges that that if you believe that you have a substance abuse problem to seek a professional's help. This book is not designed, nor is intended, to replace the advice, treatment, or programs advised to you by a health care professional. This book is designed to supplement your individual treatment program.

To find a treatment facility in your area, please visit the Substance Abuse and Mental Health Services Administration (US Department of Human Services) web site at http://findtreatment.samhsa.gov

Table of Contents

INTRODUCTION

How to use this workbook

If you are an addict, you need help. To begin to get help, you need to decide to change, but more about this, later. For now, you are looking at this workbook. So, you need some ideas about how to use it.

This workbook is yours. You should use it in ways that benefit you. To get the most benefit from it, here are some suggestions:

Take your time

Rushing through this workbook is not needed. Your recovery from addiction is not a contest. It is your pursuit of health. So, take your time, trying to make sure that you get what you need from this workbook.

Take things in order

Skipping parts of the workbook so that you can get to parts that appeal more to you will not work very well for you. If you are like most of us, we want to get to the end—to the good parts. To benefit most from the workbook, though, you need to work through each part as it comes. Some of the more challenging parts are likely the ones that will help you most.

Keep your needs in mind

As you proceed through this workbook, you need to remember that the workbook is intended to benefit you. Naturally, if you raise your level of health, you will benefit others. However, you will not likely get much from this workbook if you are doing it for others. Your recovery is rightly centered in your needs and no one else's. So, stay alert to your need for growth and health, not theirs. As you gain in health, you will find ways to benefit others, including those who are most important to you, but for now you should pay attention to your need for recovery.

Stay open to possibilities.

Once you begin to work to overcome your addiction, you will change in many ways. Some of your changes will be welcome ones and somewhat easy. Others will be stressful, confusing, and unwelcome. At this time, your decision to overcome your addiction stands on your expectation that your changes will be good ones and that the further you go, the easier your life will be. The fact is that you cannot know this, in advance of making changes. Fortunately, you don't have to know this. Luckily, for you, your will make gains for yourself, if you stay open to possibilities. Your addiction has closed many possibilities for you. One of the worst mistakes that recovering addicts make is that they try to control the process of change, just like they have tried to control their lives in other ways. Sadly, this usually prevents them from overcoming their addictions. So, Stay open to possibilities.

Full Life

Full life? Yes, full life.

If you are addicted to alcohol or drugs, you don't have a full life.

If you are addicted to alcohol or drugs, you already know what it's like to live in a way that dishonors life and that causes pain. If you have dishonored life through living as an addict, you know more than anyone else how very much you miss living a full life. You know how you have misled yourself. You know how many persons you have hurt and possibly driven away from you. You know how little joy you have. You know how empty your soul is, leaving you feeling distant from God. You know how remote from life you feel. You know the emptiness of many of your relationships. You know how much money and time you have lost from your life. You know all of this and much more, if you are an addict.

So, what it is that you have lacked, because of your addiction? Full life.

Full life is a good life. This sounds like something that may be too simple. Full life is a good life, but it is far from simple.

At the heart of full life is living honestly, as a flawed human being. This means that you are loveable and loving, willing to give

~Full Life Page 2 ~

all you have and to receive all you need. It means that you are willing and committed to receive the best that others have to offer you, knowing that you cannot adequately repay them, but it also means that you are willing to give to others, knowing that you will not receive repayment for what you give. This is full life. But there is more.

Full life means that you grow and change. If you grow and change, you become someone who is likely to be better tomorrow than you were yesterday, but it also means that living in the here-and-now is more and more possible. Obviously, being an addict takes you in the other direction, away from being better and away from living in the here-and-now, because you have lived for the next drink or the next time you can use your drug-of-choice. If you grow and change, you become a better friend to yourself. Strangely, this means that as you change, you gain an ability to manage you life. Instead of linking the parts of your life with episodes of using your addictive substance, you become free to select the better parts of your life and to cherish them. More than this, though, you become a better member of your family and a better friend.

Full life means that you live comfortably with your need for God and with a willingness to commit to God. Following scriptures, true life means that you "love God with all your heart, mind, body and soul." Most of this workbook is built around ways that you can find spiritual recovery through you mind, heart, body, and soul. But there is more.

Full life means that necessary pain is carried with honor and faith. It means that joy comes to you more readily than it ever could when you were an addict. When joy comes more readily, life is fuller than it was when you were an addict. It is full of joy, because it is also full of people who love you, along with wholeness of your mind, heart, body, and spirit. But there is more.

Full life means that you share. After all, if you live a full life, you have resources that you can share. If you life an empty life— the life of an addict—you have nothing to share. The way you share will come from your recovered life. Who knows what this may be for you? This is for you to discover. It may be helping homeless persons. It may be teaching a Sunday School class. It may be helping others to recover from their addictions. At the beginning of your recovery, you need to know only that you need to recover from your addiction. Your opportunity for service will come, later.

The Face of Spiritual Recovery

Addicts don't like to believe that they are like everyone else—vulnerable, flawed, struggling, and more. But they are like everyone else in many ways. By the time they recognize that they are addicts, they usually see their similarities with others in negative ways. However, if you are an addict, you need to recognize that you are very much like everyone else in positive ways, too.

At this time, you may not see the positive aspects of yourself, because you are an addict.

You need to understand, though, that addiction is not a natural condition, let alone a necessary one. Addiction is a disease that can be effectively managed. This means that you may anticipate a day when you are no longer an active addict. You can look forward to physical health, but also spiritual health. Helping you to find spiritual health is the aim of this workbook. This gives a serious burden to the author. Specifically, the author should give you clear, reasonable, and achievable ideas about what spiritual recovery means and how your life may be different for you as you participate in recovery.

In other words, before you begin this workbook, it should answer the question, "If you recover spiritually, what will be different for you?"

Some of the answers to this question appear below. As you read these answers, you need to keep in mind that you should see most of these signs of spiritual recovery in your recovery, but not in ways that look just like everyone else's. Your recovery will be unique, even if you share many qualities of your recovery with others.

Here are some of the common qualities of spiritual recovery. You may expect to see most of them in your recovery.

Self-awareness

If nothing else, recovery involves heightened self-awareness. The process of recovery requires you to look carefully at yourself and to see new—both good and bad—parts of yourself. A feature of your recovery is that your heightened self-awareness leads to the increasing possibility that you will also be more aware of your relationship with your Higher Power.

In the early stages of your recovery, your self-examination is likely to make you uncomfortable. This is a part of the process of gaining the self-awareness that you will need, to function well as a recovering person. Your discomfort will fade into your past, as you grow as a person. Your self-awareness, though, will stay with you and continue to bring you benefits.

Also, as you commit to spiritual growth, you will very likely also commit to carefully examining yourself so that you may continue to grow. This, too, may be uncomfortable for you, but it is necessary. Self-examination and spiritual growth should be thought of as processes that go on and on and not as achievements that end. So long as you are alive, there is no graduation from life. Life is for living. Self-examination and spiritual growth are parts of living.

Direction and purpose

Addicts have direction and purpose. Unfortunately, their direction and purpose are usually self-destructive. With recovery, though, your direction and purpose will change. For one thing, you will want to be alive, instead of feeling the dread that each day will bring another irresistible compulsion to find your drug—or poison—of choice. In your recovery, your discovery of your new direction and purpose will bring you enjoyment and demands. For you, this may be a renewed dedication to your family. Or, it may be an intensified commitment to God. Or, it may be the contentment that comes with long-time recovery and your heartfelt commitment to maintain your contentment. All of these things are yet to be discovered.

Worship

Your heightened self-awareness will give you a capacity to renew your ability to look outside yourself. This means that you will take a fresh look at your family and how you care for them. It means that you will pay with more enjoyment. It means that you will have a higher interest in helping others. However, in talking about your spiritual gains, it should be said that you will likely look outside yourself and find meaning in God—or another Higher Power. One of the common expressions of this will be your new interest worship. With recovery, you will likely have a new ability to give attention to God in a worshipful attitude.

Intimacy

In recovery, you will be much less afraid of being exposed or "found out" as an addict or just a bad person. Once this fear is gone, among the results of your recovery, you will discover—or re-discover—your ability to get close to others in a special and personal way. This means that you will find ways to care more effectively for others, but also that you will let yourself be cared for more effectively.

Heightened ability to stay sober

Your recovery will bring a degree of freedom that you may have lacked as an active addict. This comes from your increased ability to stay sober. The longer you stay sober, the more you exercise your will power to stay sober and healthy.

But there is more to this than staying sober. Surely, staying sober is absolutely necessary, if you are to maintain your health. By depending on your health—instead of your addiction—you will gain confidence in life as good and in yourself as a person with wisdom and good judgment.

A little more about your freedom needs to be said. Once you are no longer dependent on your addictive substance, you will have gained a lot of personal freedom. With your freedom, you will carry a large responsibility for deciding what to do with your freedom. For many individuals in recovery, freedom becomes a way to pursue spiritual development and to connect with God.

The addicted ego wants to tie itself to habits that are self-destructive. The healthy ego wants to connect itself to others who are healthy and to God, the giver of life and health. The healthy ego wants to live gratefully, peacefully, and generously. In this, there is freedom that is refreshing and inviting.

Serenity and mental focus

With recovery, you will develop calmness. Instead of living with the dread that your life is bad and getting worse because of your addiction, you will worry less about your future and function more effectively in your daily life. Some of this comes because you feel increasingly better about your growing record of sobriety. With your record of sobriety—and the clean mind and heart that comes with sobriety--you will develop spiritually, including developing serenity and mental focus.

The fact is that clean thoughts and clean feelings go together. However, the longer you have clean thoughts and feelings, you become less focused on yourself and increasingly capable of letting God enter your life.

Service

As you continue in your recovery, you will very likely decide to be helpful to others who need you. You will likely act on behalf of others, with no expectation of getting anything from your actions, except gratitude for having the personal resources that you can use to benefit others.

Many individuals in recovery decide to mentor others who need the help that comes from someone with more experience in recovery. So, as you live in recovery for a long period of time, you will have experience that will be useful to others who are early in their recovery. Because others helped you in your recovery, you will probably want to help "give back" to those who helped you.

Humility

Along with recovery, a debt comes to you. If you are beginning your recovery, don't worry about a debt that may come to you in the future. Your recovery is more important than anticipating a debt.

The fact is, though, the longer you live in recovery and have received life-saving help from others, you will feel a debt of gratitude. And, gratitude comes from thinking of the seriousness of the gifts that you have received, not from self-serving pride. This is the heart of humility. As others have said, "humility is not thinking less of yourself, but thinking of yourself less."

The great thing about thinking of yourself less is that you are left open to receiving even more from those who care about you. So, instead of simply taking credit for your good life in recovery, you will find that your humility can connect you with others and with God, without your ego getting in the way. This allows you to think more of others and their welfare.

Connection with a community

The recovery community is a large one. As a recovering person, you will be a part of it. This is something to look forward to.

As you look forward to being a part of the recovery community, you may need to know that it is held together by love. Even when the members of the recovery don't speak a lot about love, it is love that holds it together. Love is the life-affirming and driving force that enables the members of the recovery community to help addicts re-gain lives that are healthy and spiritually alive. In this community, you will learn that love can be delivered in a selfless and enthusiastic way. You will learn that you can live in harmony with others, with yourself, and with God, because you will see many others doing this.

Beliefs that will give you meaning

As you seek recovery and live in recovery, you will gain beliefs that you will carry with you for the rest of your life. Only you can determine what these beliefs will be. However, many recovering individuals list the things that are included in this discussion. They include a belief in the goodness of others. They include a belief in the soundness of your own judgment, free of your addiction. They include a belief in the power of a community through which addicts can re-gain their health. They include a belief in a Higher Power. And much more.

Joy

Addicts are not happy. In recovery, recovering addicts do more than lose their addictions. Usually, they re-gain enjoyment of life.

Most individuals want to be happy. Addicts learn that they may be happy—even joyful—by appreciating their lives in recovery. Instead of killing themselves with their addictive substances, they live in freedom. Instead of denying their most important personal needs for love, family, and more, they enjoy love and family. And much more.

Obviously, joy is not a certainty for anyone. Living in freedom from addictive substances, though, dramatically increases the possibility of happiness.

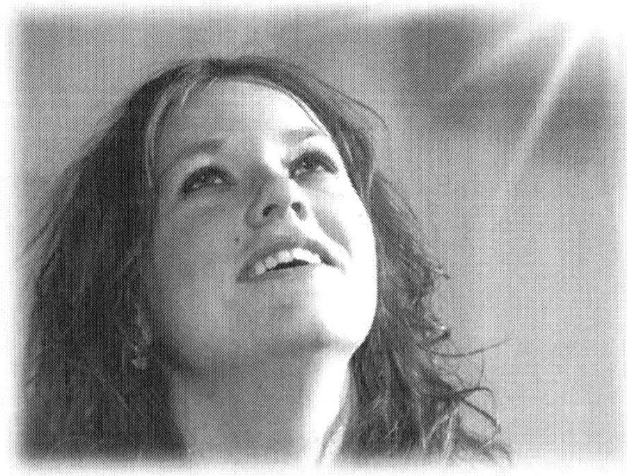

GETTING STARTED

Deciding

If you are reading this, you know that you need to change. Reading this, though, cannot make you change.

The fact is that only you can decide to get rid of your addiction to alcohol or drugs. Without your decision to change, nothing happens.

Deciding to free yourself from your addiction is not easy, but freeing yourself from your addiction is very much better than dying with your addiction. Deciding to change is the beginning of change. Without your decision to change, you won't change. So, what have you decided? Are you ready to begin the process of change? If you are ready to begin the process of change, please proceed through this workbook.

And, welcome to your start toward freedom from addictions and freedom to gain a full life for yourself.

Support

If you have decided to change—to get rid of your addiction—you will need all of the help you can get. The best evidence says that those who have the support of others are more likely to succeed than those who lack support from others. The truth is that it is one thing to suffer through recovery alone and another thing entirely to suffer through recovery with support from others. Your suffering, though, is not the complete story of recovery. The complete story includes the joy of recovery that you find by rediscovering your useful and positive interest in living and finding real love in your relationships, and a meaningful relationship with God. When this happens, your suffering remains real, but much less important.

If you have decided to change—to recover from your addiction—and to seek a full life, you need to get to work. So, your first task it to list those whom you can count on. Who are they? What can you expect of each one?

What Can I Expect From This Person

Please add pages, if you need more space than this.

Personal Assets

As you work to recover from your addiction, you may believe that you are beginning your work with no strength or personal assets. Probably, this is not true. While you may understandably feel weak, with little working for you, you bring values and other personal assets that will help you to recover.

So, your next assignment is to identify the personal assets that may help you to recover. Another way to think about this assignment is that you are an addict, but there is much more to being you than being an addict. The assignment helps you to identify some important parts of yourself that your addiction has not killed.

The following lists of personal assets are ones that others have identified. You may notice how different they are. Yours will be different from theirs.

Person One	**Person Two**	**Person Three**
Hopeful	Religious	Honest
Loving	Spiritual	Disciplined
Family	Generous	Strong
Curious	Compassionate	Faithful
Optimistic	Worshipful	Cooperative
Aggressive	Gallant	Confident
Honest	Spontaneous	Spiritual
Industrious	Patriotic	Loving
Respectful	Realistic	Religious
Family oriented	Loving	Persuasive

Obviously, your assets may be different from the ones above. For example, the persons above did not list "healthy" or "intelligent" or "ethical," as one of their assets.

Listing your assets may be easy. In fact, all you need to do, for now, is to just list them. As you proceed through this section, you will have an opportunity to do more with them. For now, though, you need to create your own list of your personal assets.

The list of personal assets, below, is intended only to make suggestions. Your personal assets are not necessarily on the list. As you read the list, make a record of the ones that fit you best, by writing them in the empty column on the right side of the page. For now, you are the only one who is making the list and who will read it. Quite possibly, you will be the only person who ever sees it. This is up to you.

Also, please remember that you may have personal assets that do not appear on the list.

The list of your personal assets may include more items than the number of blanks provided. Please, write any additional assets in the margins. Make a record of all of the assets that you believe fit you at this time.

Please, record your personal assets in the column on the right side of the page.

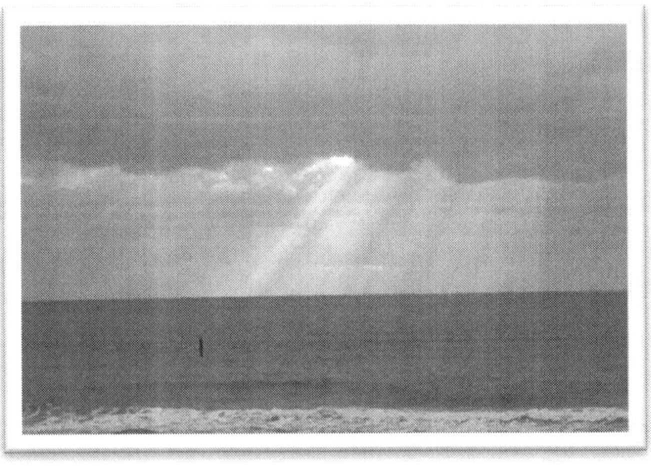

Accepting	Accomplished	Accountable	______________
Accurate	Active	Adaptable	______________
Adventuring	Affectionate	Aggressive	______________
Agile	Alert	Altruistic	______________
Ambitious	Amusing	Approachable	______________
Assertive	Attentive	Attractive	______________
Beautiful	Benevolent	Bold	______________
Brave	Calm	Candid	______________
Capable	Careful	Caring	______________
Charming	Cheerful	Clean	______________
Cleverness	Collaborative	Comforting	______________
Compassionate	Communicative	Compassionate	______________
Competent	Competitive	Confident	______________
Congruent	Content	Cooperative	______________
Coordinated	Cordial	Courageous	______________
Courteous	Creative	Credible	______________
Cunning	Curious	Daring	______________
Decisive	Delightful	Democratic	______________
Dependable	Determined	Devout	______________
Diligent	Disciplined	Dutiful	______________
Educated	Effective	Efficient	______________
Elegant	Empathic	Energetic	______________

Encouraging	Ethical	Exciting	_________________
Extroverted	Fair	Family oriented	_________________
Famous	Fearless	Gallant	_________________
Generous	Gentle	Giving	_________________
Good	Gracious	Grateful	_________________
Gregarious	Growing	Faithful	_________________
Ferocious	Friendly	Frugal	_________________
Fun	Hard working	Healthy	_________________
Helpful	Hopeful	Honest	_________________
Honorable	Heroic	Holy	_________________
Humble	Humorous	Hygienic	_________________
Imaginative	Independent	Industrious	_________________
Insightful	Inspirational	Intelligent	_________________
Introverted	Intuitive	Inventive	_________________
Judicious	Just	Kind	_________________
Knowledgeable	Logical	Loving	_________________
Loyal	Mature	Meek	_________________
Meticulous	Modest	Moral	_________________
Neat	Obedient	Open	_________________
Optimistic	Orderly	Ordinary	_________________
Organized	Passionate	Patriotic	_________________
Peaceful	Persistent	Persuasive	_________________

Pious	Playful	Poised	__________
Positive	Powerful	Practical	__________
Prayerful	Productive	Progressive	__________
Prosperous	Prudent	Punctual	__________
Quick	Realistic	Reasonable	__________
Reliable	Religious	Resilient	__________
Respectful	Resourceful	Responsible	__________
Reverent	Romantic	Sacrificial	__________
Self-reliant	Sensual	Serene	__________
Serving	Sharing	Shrewd	__________
Silly	Simple	Sincere	__________
Skillful	Spiritual	Spontaneous	__________
Stable	Strong	Successful	__________
Supportive	Thrifty	Tolerant	__________
Traditional	Trustworthy	Truthful	__________
Unique	Wholesome	Wise	__________
Witty	Worshipful	Virtuous	__________
Visionary	Zealous		__________

The next step in identifying your personal assets is to select the ten that you believe represent you most accurately. From the list above, write the assets that most accurately represent you on the blanks below. For now, do not be concerned about which ones may be more important than the others. Just list the ones that accurately represent you.

____

____

____

____

____

____

____

____

Now, to determine your most important assets, use the spaces below to list the ten assets that most accurately represent you. Try to list them in their order of importance, with "1" being the most important to you.

1. __________________________

2. __________________________

3. __________________________

4. __________________________

5. __________________________

6. __________________________

7. __________________________

8. __________________________

9. __________________________

10. __________________________

You have more work to do with your list of assets. You need to identify actions that indicate how you use your assets. What specific actions illustrate how you use your assets?

For example, if you list "Generous," in what ways are you generous? Do you give your time in volunteer service? Do you give your money to causes in which you believe, such as the American Red Cross, the Salvation Army, or Habitat for Humanity? What do you do with your assets? The blank chart below provides space for only ten assets.

<u>YOUR ASSETS</u>
    <u>THE WAYS YOU PRACTICE YOUR ASSETS</u>

1. ___________________

____

____

2. ________________

____

____

3. ______________

____

____

4. ______________

____

____

5. ______________

____

____

6. ______________

____

____

7. ________________________

____

____

8. ________________________

____

____

9. ________________________

____

____

10. ________________________

____

____

You are not yet finished with work on your personal assets. The next step is to eliminate all but the five of your most important personal assets. Place them in the blanks below.

1. ________________________   My most important asset

2. ________________________

3. ________________________

4. ________________________

5. ________________________

This short list of your personal assets gives you a snapshot of what is most important to you. Your last task here is to describe what your addiction has done to your most important personal assets. This exercise may require you to test your honesty and your imagination. It asks you to think about some of the consequences of your addiction. In particular, it asks you to answer the question, "What has your addiction done to your ability to use your most important personal assets?" Write your answer in the space below.

____

____

____

____

____

____

____

____

____

____

____

THE STEPS

The rest of your workbook is based on The Twelve Steps. The twelve steps come from the tradition of Alcoholics Anonymous. However, the steps are presented in a fresh and inviting manner here. They are alive, just as you are. In their original form, here are the Twelve Steps:

1. We admitted we were powerless over alcohol—that our lives had become unmanageable.

2. Came to believe that a Power greater than ourselves could restore us to sanity.

3. Made a decision to turn our will and our lives over to the care of God as we understood Him.

4. Made a searching and fearless moral inventory of ourselves.

5. Admitted to God, to ourselves, and to another human being the exact nature of our wrongs.

6. Were entirely ready to have God remove all these defects of character.

7. Humbly asked Him to remove our shortcomings.

8. Made a list of all persons we had harmed, and became willing to make amends to them all.

9. Made direct amends to such people wherever possible, except when to do so would injure them or others.

10. Continued to take personal inventory and when we were wrong promptly admitted it.

11. Sought through prayer and meditation to improve our conscious contact with God as we understood Him, praying only for knowledge of His will for us and the power to carry that out.

12. Having had a spiritual awakening as the result of these steps, we tried to carry this message to others, and to practice these principles in all our affairs.

The Twelve Steps may be compared to the twelve hours on the face of a clock, with each of the steps being steps being matched with each of the hours of the clock. If you think of the twelve steps as the hours on the clock, you may begin to think that the steps may be repeated many times. This is the idea. Just as every day brings one o'clock in the afternoon, all of us who seek to recover from addictions need to face—again and again—the issue of step one—our powerlessness—and learn more about our way of managing our powerlessness each time we face it. So, as you work your way through each of the twelve steps, you may want to review the ones that you have already completed. Actually, after you have completed all of the steps, you will want to work through them again, so that you may be able to remember and take advantage of the gains that you have achieved.

This is another way of saying that recovery is a life-long process. Recovery is growth toward health. It doesn't stop. So, just like the time of day—one o'clock in the afternoon—recovery needs to be seen as something that challenges us every day. To put this in other words, if we lived in a healthy manner yesterday, we need to renew the commitment to live in a healthy manner today and every day that comes.

Here are the 12 steps of recovery and the hours of the day:

STEP	HOUR	AREA OF GROWTH
Step One	1 O'clock	Admitting powerlessness
Step Two	2 O'clock	Acknowledging Greater Power
Step Three	3 O'clock	Making a decision
Step Four	4 O'clock	Taking inventory
Step Five	5 O'clock	Admitting to God
Step Six	6 O'clock	Ready to change
Step Seven	7 O'clock	Humbly asking
Step Eight	8 O'clock	Making a list
Step Nine	9 O'clock	Making amends
Step Ten	10 O'clock	Continue taking inventory
Step Eleven	11O'clock	Prayer and meditation
Step Twelve	12 O'clock	Spiritual awakening

To assist you in remembering the steps and the hours, your next task is to write each

AREA OF GROWTH by its hour on the face of the clock below.

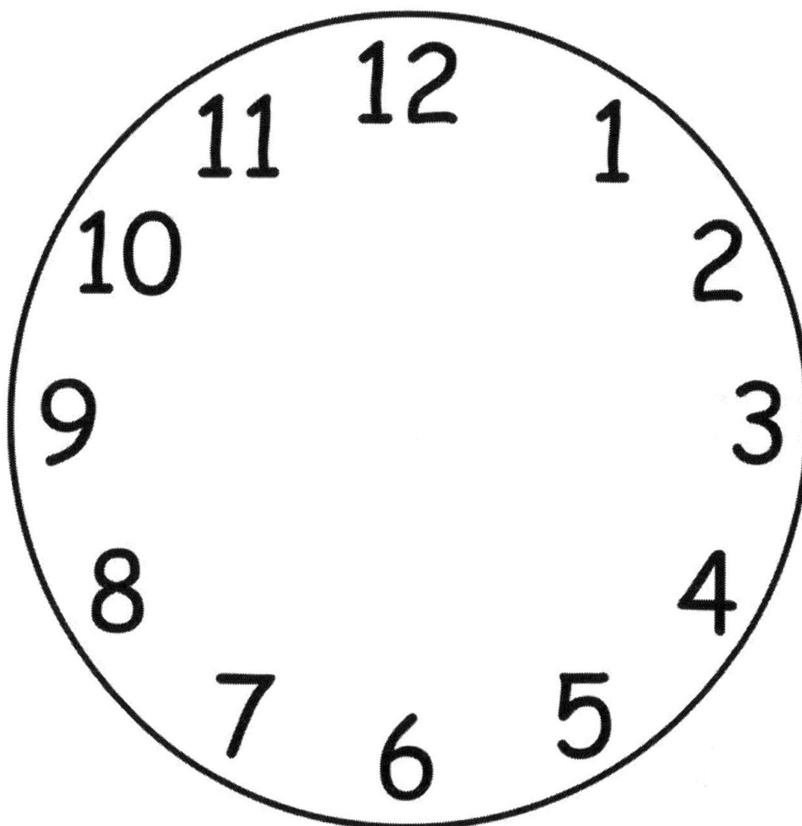

All of the steps and hours in this workbook include the same parts. One part is a prayer. The prayer is given with the idea that you may need some assistance in shaping your thoughts, as you seek spiritual growth. Also, you will be asked to write your own prayer in each of the steps.

Another part is a lesson. The lesson in each step is provided so that you may be able to gain some understanding of the step and the areas of growth that may be important for you. As you read the lesson, you should ask yourself about the ways that you can take advantage of the lesson. You may want to add your thoughts to the lesson. For this purpose, space is provided at the end of the lesson.

Another part is an exercise. The exercise asks you to make a record of your thoughts about your growth in the step. In most steps, you are asked to make a record of how your growth may be seen in your heart, mind, body, and soul. This will be challenging for you, but facing the challenges and achieving recovery is far more important than completing this workbook. It is a matter of recovering you life—a life that is worth living, for you and for others.

ONE O'CLOCK
STEP ONE
Admitting powerlessness

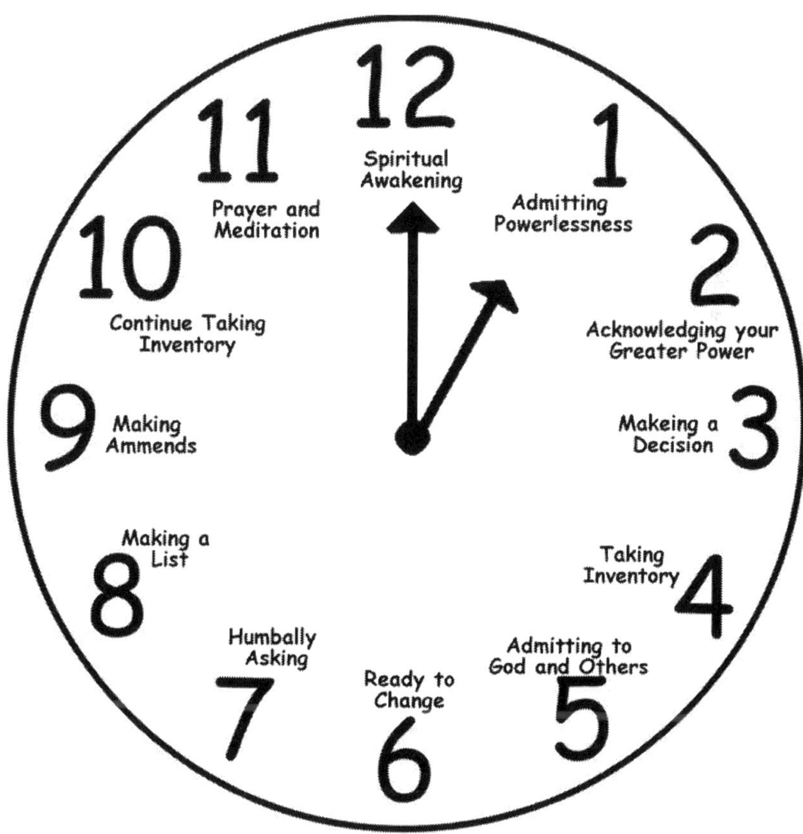

Step One says,
"We admitted we were powerless over alcohol—that our
lives had become unmanageable."

Step One Prayer

Dear Lord,

I have let alcohol take over my life. For alcohol, I have abandoned some of the things that are most important to me—family, good sense, health, faith, money, and a lot more. And, now, I am not important to them. I have failed others and have failed myself. I have no excuses for what I have done.

Lord, I have come to realize that I have let alcohol take over my life and that I have no control to manage myself. I am powerless over alcohol.

Lord, I do not like the person I have become. I am empty. Unable to find my way, I am lost. Turning to alcohol, instead of the love of people who are important to me, I am lonely. Having closed my mind and heart to health, I am sick.

Now, Lord, with little to offer to you or to those who are important to me and having lost many things that are important to me, I pray that I have everything to gain, by admitting my powerlessness. I pray that I may be able to depend on your strength, because I cannot depend on my own strength.

Lord, in this early hour of my recovery, I have a long way to go. Please, be with me. Amen.

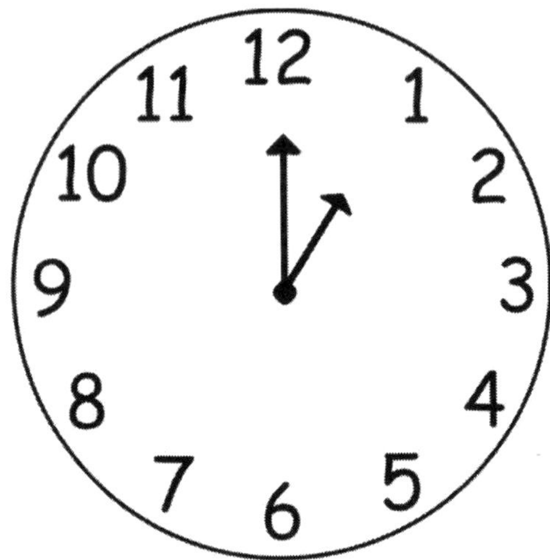

Step One Lesson
Powerlessness

Powerlessness is many things, when we experience it. It is painful. It is frustrating. It is humiliating. More than pain or frustration or humiliation, though, it is opportunity. After all, if you are powerless, everything you do from this moment forward adds to your ability to manage your life effectively and enjoyably, if you have decided to seek health for yourself.

For example, look at the mom who has become a really bad parent because of her addiction. Like most addicts, she doesn't want to admit that she is powerless over her addiction and that her addiction has made her a bad parent. It hurts too much to do this. To admit this means that she must see—really look at—the terrible damage that she has done to her children. So, she avoids admitting that she is powerless. Still, as difficult as this may be, admitting her powerlessness and the negative impact of her addiction on her children gives her freedom to change—freedom that she has not had. Once she admits her powerlessness, she acknowledges that she has failed and that she is now free to do things differently. Once she begins to be honest with herself, she can look honestly at what she has done, but also at what may be possible for her in the future. Once she honestly looks at the damage that she has done to her children, she can begin to think about how to help her children to heal. The hard thing for her, though, is the beginning— admitting that she is powerless.

If this is where you are, it is time for you to admit what you know to be true. It is time to admit that you have let your addiction take over your life.

The "blessing" below is reported to have been prayed over Henri Nouwen by his spiritual teacher and leader.

- May all your expectations be frustrated.
- May all your plans be thwarted.
- May all your desires be withered into nothingness.

- That you may experience the powerlessness and the poverty of a child and sing and dance in the love of God the Father, the Son and the Spirit.[1]

The idea here is that addicts find great freedom in admitting their powerlessness.

Admitting that you are powerless may seem to be a simple thing to do. It isn't. So, as you consider making this admission, you may want to ask yourself what this means. Here are some questions that may help you. Does powerlessness mean that you have

- Lived as if the purpose of your life is being an addict?
- Lost your ability to be creative?
- Refused to bring healthy people into your life?
- Lived as if your spiritual life did not belong to you or even exist?
- Let yourself get stuck with pessimistic thinking?
- Spent your money on your addiction, instead of important things and people?
- Wasted your health?
- Ignored the needs of your family?
- Let enjoyment of your life and others' slip away from you?
- Allowed heartache become a way of life for you?
- Avoided God?
- Emptied you mind and heart of positive meaning?
- Narrowed your view of your future to your next drink?
- Let your personal history be remembered with stained and painful pictures?
- Lost the strength to resist your addictive actions?
- Invented great but false reasons to continue your addiction?
- Acted as if your body can handle all possible punishment that you give it?

---

[1] (Nouwen)

Step One
An Exercise for You

Of course, there is more to being powerless than these questions may indicate. The questions may not match your kind of powerlessness. Your kind of powerlessness is something that you must define for yourself. What does your powerlessness look like? What does it feel like? How has it affected your heart, mind, body, and soul? Answering this question is your next assignment. In the boxes, below, write your answer. How has your addiction affected your heart, mind, body and soul?

To give you a little help with this, here are some ways that you may think about your heart, mind, body and soul.
So far, in Step One, you have read a prayer, studied a lesson, and described your powerlessness. Now, your final task in Step One is to write your prayer. Please, write your prayer about powerlessness in the space below.

Heart	Mind
refers to affection, values, attitudes, close human relationships, ambitions, and related things.	refers to thoughts, reasons, problem solving skills, beliefs, planning, and related things
Body	**Soul**
refers to energy, health, resting, sleeping, sex, nutrition, safety, and related things	refers to peace of mind, faith, meaning, spirituality, religious commitment and practices, and related things.

MY PRAYER ABOUT BEING POWERLESS

TWO O'CLOCK
STEP TWO
Acknowledging Your Greater Power

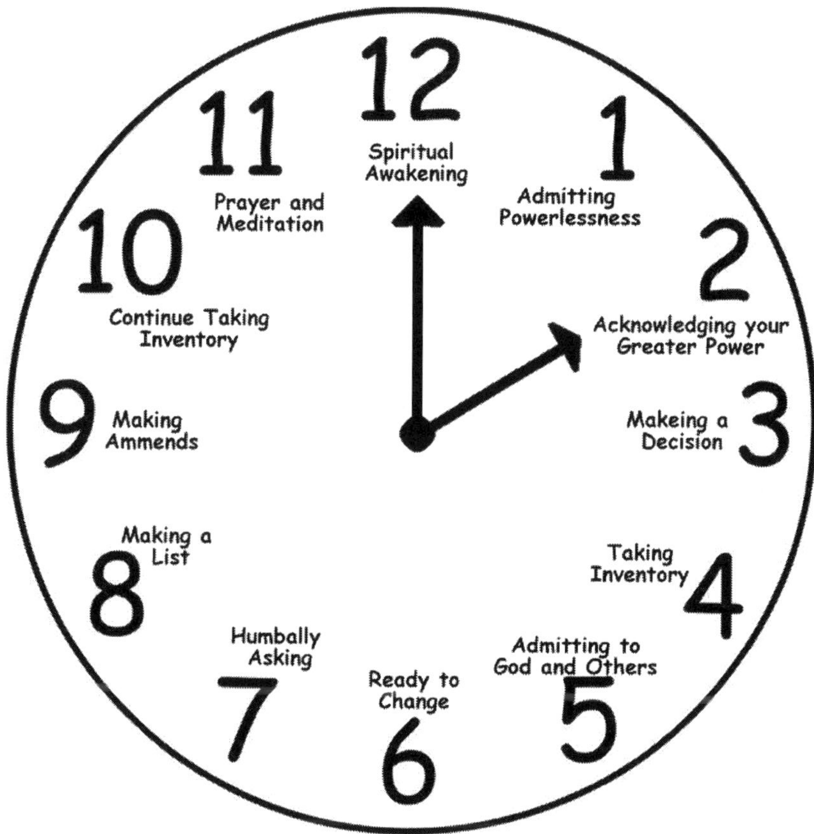

Step Two says,
"I came to believe that a Power greater than myself could restore me to sanity.

Step Two Prayer

Dear Lord,

I am stuck in my addiction. This is a dark hour for me. I am broken. I am alone. I do not have the power alone to help myself. I am helpless. I don't know anyone else who can help me, either. So, here I am, powerless and need power that I don't have. I need to depend on someone with power.

Here I am, with nothing to offer you, Lord, except to come to you with my need for you. I need you. Lord, if I can't help myself, I need you to help me. You are a Power who is much greater than I am.

My prayer is that I may be acceptable to you, that I may get close enough to you to allow you to restore me to health, that I may recover the good relationships that I have lost, and that I may receive opportunities for service.

Lord, I am uncertain about what may happen to me, but I am turning to you for direction.

Thank you, Lord.

Amen

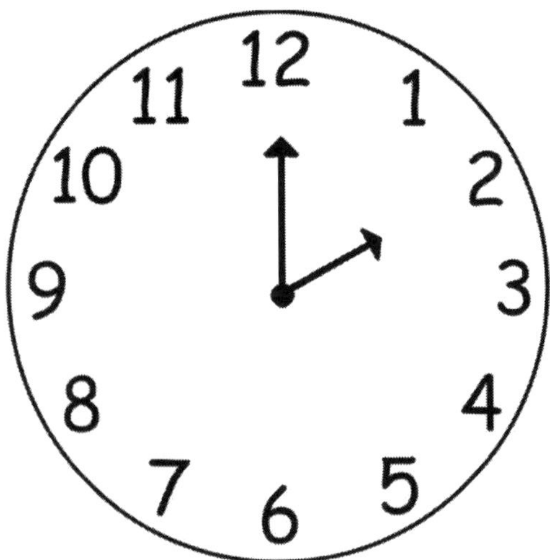

Step Two Lesson
The Need for a Higher Power

A recovering addict said, "My addiction is like being stuck in traffic when you got to get somewhere in hurry. I'm stuck. I need everything and can't get anything I need. My wife is gone. My kids won't speak to me. Why should they? I wouldn't speak to me, either, if they had done to me what I've done to them. It hurts to think about it. I look like hell. I never thought that this could happen to me. And I'm not getting anywhere. I want to let go of it, but I can't. I need help."

This is what many addicts experience. They are stuck in their addiction. They are powerless to escape the pain and destructiveness of their addiction. Because of this, they need to acknowledge that a power outside themselves may be necessary, if they are going to escape from their addiction.

If you are an addict, you question may not be one of whether you need a higher power, but one of which higher power you seek. As an addict, you need a power outside yourself.

Before you select a higher power upon which to depend, you will need to first face yourself. This comes before you select or commit to a higher power. If you are trying to escape from your addiction, while continuing to believe that you can escape on your own—your own energy, your own insight, your own management of your life, your own ability to control your recovery—you are not ready for a higher power. So, before you look to a higher power, you need to acknowledge that you are powerless and that you need someone outside yourself.

The idea that we may gain health and effective management of life through becoming powerless appears to make little sense. The idea, though, is at the heart of effective living—living so that life is known to be truly worthwhile.

Whether you are a Christian or not, you can read Jesus' Sermon on the Mount and get a picture of the importance of being powerless as a basis for depending on a higher power and a start toward recovery. In the Sermon on the Mount, Jesus began with this, "Blessed are those who know their need for God, for the Kingdom of Heaven is theirs."

The idea here is that recovery includes knowing that you need recovery and that you may not have enough personal strength to recover on your own. Based on this, as an addict, you do not have to know God, but to know your need for God. In the same way, you don't have to know how to repair teeth, but to know your need for a dentist. Knowing your need for God is the heart of Step Two. This is another sign of the beginning of your recovery—acknowledging your need for God.

You may wonder about the idea of "Blessed," as Jesus used it. Generally, the idea is that those who know their need for God are secure and happy. Clearly, the values that Jesus presented in the Sermon on the Mount are different from most Americans' values. You may want to give careful attention to these values, as you consider your Higher Power.

Our Way of Thinking	Jesus' Lessons for Us
Own as much we can buy	Blessed are those who know their as need for God, for theirs is the kingdom of heaven.
Laugh, spend, and party, frequently	Blessed are those who mourn, for they shall be comforted.
Take charge and control others	Blessed are the gentle, for they shall inherit the earth.
Seek praise, rewards, status, and money	Blessed are those who hunger and thirst for righteousness, for they shall be satisfied.
Get all you can and take no prisoners	Blessed are the merciful, for they shall receive mercy.
Know pleasure, escape from purity	Blessed are the pure in heart, for they shall see God.

Our Way of Thinking	Jesus' Lessons for Us
Gain possessions, not peace or peace of mind	Blessed are the peacemakers, for they shall be called sons of God.
Pleasure, now! Not persecution or righteousness	Blessed are those who have been persecuted for the sake of for theirs is the kingdom of heaven.
Jesus? Jesus is good, he helps me to get what I want.	Blessed are you when people insult if you and persecute you, and falsely say all kinds of evil against you because of Me.

When you acknowledge your need for a Higher Power, you acknowledge your need to change, to move toward a different way of living. With this, you have to wonder what this may require of you. In other words, what may a higher power look like? Here are some possibilities:

Your Higher Power will have a position of real importance in your life. You don't need just another token of commitment. This is a life-and-death matter, not one of convenience.

Your Higher Power will be a source of positive direction for you. This may be seen in the Sermon on the Mount, above. However, it may be seen in many other ways, whether you are a Christian, a Native American, a Muslim, or a devotee of most other major religious orientations.

Your Higher Power will expect active commitment from you and will be a source of meaning for you. This means that you will need to be an active player in your recovery and that your Higher Power will be a source if meaning, inspiration, direction, advice, and community. In other words, you give to and you get from your Higher Power.

Your Higher Power will be a source of specific insight. This may be seen in the Sermon on the Mount. For example, the idea that knowing your need for God may be a forecast of spiritual reward is an important insight.

Your Higher Power will be a source of new information. Along with inspiration and insight, you will gain new information. This may be information that lets you know that you can move toward recovery from your addiction. For example, many approaches to spirituality require the practice of certain disciplines. Usually, these disciplines involve regular schedules of practice, such as a regular time for prayer or meditation. Having this information may be helpful for you.

Your Higher Power will help you to find new and better standards of behavior. This may mean that you will find ways to share your personal resources with others. It may mean that you hear of ways to change, such as learning about specific reading from which others have gained or a schedule for prayer that has helped others.

Your Higher Power will help you to acquire meaningful rewards. Based on the experience of many others who have lived in recovery, this may mean that you will gain positive and enduring personal relationships, both in the recovery community and elsewhere. It may mean that you will find a spiritual community that contributes to your life long after you are sober and clean. It may mean that you find rewarding opportunities for service, because you will have a great deal to share as a recovering individual.

Step Two
An Exercise for You

This exercise is your opportunity to think about your Higher Power. It is used here because, if you maintain your recovery, you will need to be clear about how you think about your Higher Power. Keep in mind, though, that the information that you provide here may be changed as you continue with your recovery. For now, before making any commitments—except for the commitment to recover—you need to think about your Higher Power.

The exercise is simple, but challenging. Your task is to write a word for each letter in the words, "H-I-G-H-E-R P-O-W-E-R." For example, for the letter "H," you may want to write "Helper." Write words that best fit your idea about what your Higher Power means to you. Don't be concerned about whether anyone else may approve of your words. They are yours. They are intended to help you clarify your thinking about your Higher Power.

<u>Letter</u> **<u>First Choice</u>**   **<u>Other Word</u>**

H ______________________   ______________________

I ______________________   ______________________

G ______________________   ______________________

H ______________________   ______________________

E ______________________   ______________________

R ______________________   ______________________

P ______________________   ______________________

O ______________________   ______________________

W ______________________   ______________________

E ______________________   ______________________

R ______________________   ______________________

Now that you have assigned words to your Higher Power, take this exercise a little further. As you study your selection of words, what do you know about your view of your Higher Power? What does your Higher Power mean to you? Write your answers in the space below.

____

____

____

____

____

____

____

____

____

____

____

THREE O'CLOCK
STEP THREE:
Making a decision

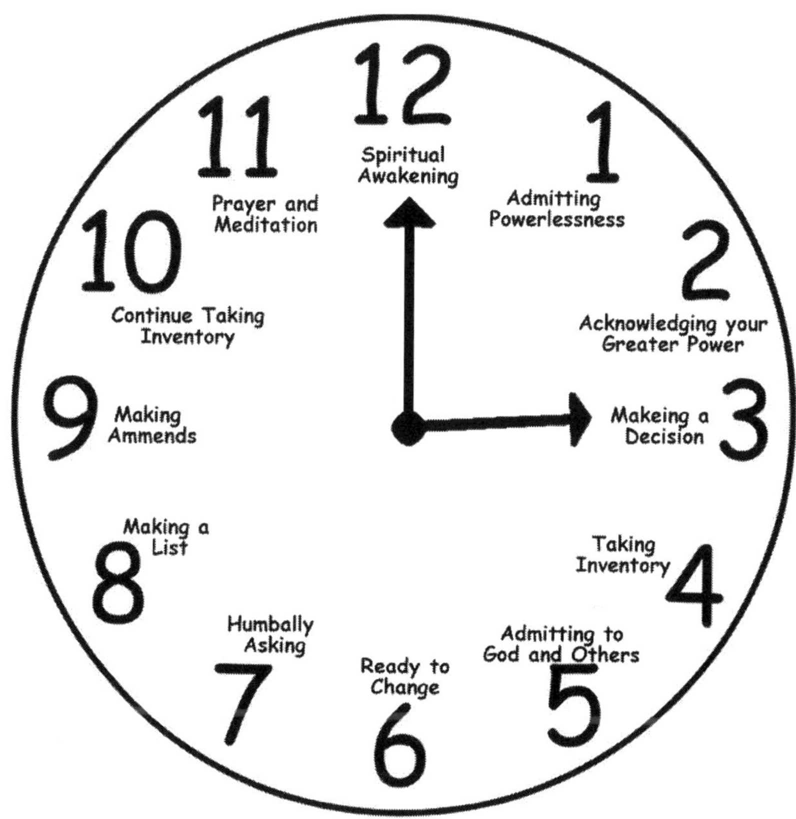

Step Three says,
"Made a decision to turn our will and our lives over to the
care of God as we understood Him."

Step Three Prayer

Dear Lord,

My addiction has taken me down a long, muddy road. My shoes are covered with mud. I can hardly walk. My head is full of crazy ideas, muddy just like my shoes. I have convinced myself that I can make it on my own. That's a muddy idea. I have talked myself into thinking that I can quit my addiction any time I want to. That's another muddy idea. I have convinced myself that I can really enjoy my addiction, that my addicted friends are good for me, and that my family will stay with me, no matter how much I hurt them. Those are all muddy ideas.

My thinking is so bad that even I can't stand it.

I'm too tired to go on. I have no peace of mind. I have let my health slip away. I have neglected my real friends. I have failed my family. I can't make it on my own. I can't quit my addiction without help. My thinking is so bad that even I can't stand it.

Here I am. Standing here in the mud. I can't go on like this. My mind is filthy. My thinking is so bad that even I can't stand it.

Lord, thank you, because I am not dead, yet. Please, help me to restore sobriety and health.

Now, I need a hand. I need to get out of my filth and into my faith. I need to find my life, again. I need you in my life. This is everything to me, right now.

Amen.

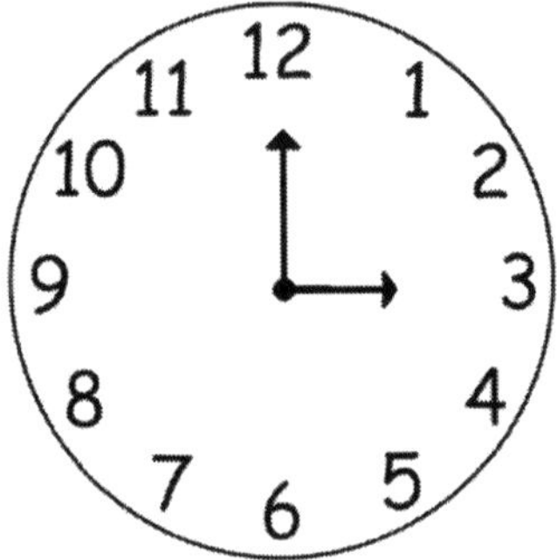

Step Three Lesson
Making a Decision

Making a decision to seek health is harder than it seems. If you are an addict, the fact is that you have been making decisions that have hurt you and others, for a long time now. So, why should you do things differently, now that you are disappointed, if not disgusted, with yourself? Probably, you have been disappointed and disgusted for quite a while, now.

Clearly, you wish to escape from the imprisonment of your addiction. Making the decision to escape from your imprisonment requires more than a wish to get away from it. It requires you to acknowledge that you cannot make it on your own and that you turn your will and life to the care of God as you understand God.

Once you have turned to God, you must develop specific plans for your recovery. The rest of this workbook intends to help you to develop your recovery plan.

For now, though, you need to make a decision to commit your will and life to God. So, what could possibly get in the way of your decision? Here are some thoughts about this.

Those who are addicts do not want to understand their addiction. Further, they really want to deny the seriousness of their problems. After all, facing the problems requires honesty and the pain that comes from honesty. Then, as if this were not enough, addicts usually do not want to give up their addiction—one of the few things in their lives that they want to believe helps them to feel good. Giving up this belief exposes the addict to unwanted consequences. One of these consequences is that the exposure of the addict's irrational beliefs that addicts fuel with their poisonous substances. Another is the exposure of the addict's waste of health, money, and persons they love. Maybe, worst of all, though, is the exposure of the addict's stupidity, foolishness, and shame. Of course, another likely consequence is that recovering addicts have to face other persons whom they have hurt. So, addicts feel a lot of pressure to avoid making a decision to get sober and healthy.

Although making the decision to get sober and healthy may be an anguished one, the outcome of not making it is ongoing decline and probably death.

However, as an addict, you must reckon with the fact that the consequences of your addiction are things about which you already know. Your irrational beliefs are not new to you. Your waste of people and money is not new to you. Your stupidity, foolishness, and shame are not new to you. The fact is that in making your decision to get sober and healthy, you will not likely discover things about yourself that are much worse than what you know already. Still, although you know these things, truly accepting them as yours is painful and challenging. Accepting the pain and challenge is the beginning of your decision, because this is a way of saying, "I am an addict."

"I am an addict." This acceptance gives you a foundation upon which to build your recovery. It says that you recognize your condition. With this recognition, you can explore your condition and receive ways to change.

The other part of Step Three is that your decision is to turn your will and life over to your Higher Power. This requires you to change directions in your thinking and in your heart and soul.

You need to consider what this may mean. It means that you are willing to change and that you bring an open mind to your need to change. It means that you are willing to examine your old attitudes and to change them. It means that you are willing to acknowledge your addictive mistakes and habits and that you replace them with spiritual practices. You will learn more about spiritual practices, later.

These things sound pretty good, don't they? You need take these things further, though. Your willingness to change and to replace your addictive habits with spiritual practices means that your will is no longer as important as it was. Obviously, your ability to fix yourself is a doubtful one. So, as to turn your will and life over to your Higher Power your will gets smaller. Your self-centeredness is no longer needed. Once you turn to your Higher Power, you give yourself to your Higher Power, including your pain, your addiction, and your disappointments, along with your day-to-day concerns.

In all of these things, you may begin to get a glimpse of hope for you. The glimpse of hope comes from the fact that you have begun to get honest about your addiction and have begun to change because you are honest. A necessary feature of your honest is to admit that there is a power that is higher than yours. Even with this, though, you need to clarify your personal understanding of what your higher power means to you. To help you to do this, you will find an exercise later in the material about Step Three.

Your understanding of your Higher Power must come from you. Your understanding of your Higher Power may look a lot like the Higher Power of others, but yours must be yours, not theirs. This is the God of your understanding, not theirs. This is the God to whom you offer prayers, not theirs.

The material here assumes that God is the God of the Christian tradition. However, for you, this may not work. Your God must be something in which you can place your faith. For you, this may be the God of the Christian tradition or the God of another religious tradition. However, it may be something else that is very different from this kind of God. It may be your childhood home. It may be your selected place in nature, such as a tree or your special place to be alone with nature. It may be your memory of the best person you have ever known.

The point is that you need to be able to relate and pray to your Higher Power according to your understanding of your Higher Power. Also, you need remember that your ongoing recovery may require you to change your Higher Power. As you grow in recovery, you may need a Higher Power that is different from the one with which you began your recovery.

You may want to think of your Higher Power as someone with whom you would be willing to leave your wallet or purse, your checkbook, or your child. This involves trust and dependability. But it also involves your faith in the one with whom you would leave these things.

Your understanding of your Higher Power should be one that expects good things from you. At least, your Higher Power should expect recovery from your addiction. But more than this, your Higher Power should expect you to act in mature, reasonable, responsible, and healthy ways. In this kind of understanding, you will find the beginning of hope, including hope for recovery.

Step Three Exercises

There are three exercises for your work on Step Three. One asks you to look at your decision making. Another asks you to examine your understanding of your Higher Power

YOUR DECISION MAKING

Have you made a decision to turn your will and your life over to your Higher Power?

(circle one)

Yes   or   No

Did you make your decision on your own, with no inappropriate pressure?

(circle one)

Yes   or   No

What issues did you consider in making your decision?

____

____

____

____

____

____

____

In turning your will over to your Higher Power, what is it that you
are turning over?

If others helped you to make your decision about turning your life
over to your Higher Power, how did they help and what would you
want them to know about your decision?

Before making your decision to turn your life over to your Higher
Power, what was your relationship with your Higher Power?

____

____

____

____

____

____

Describe the times you felt the presence of your Higher Power
while you were using your addictive substance.

____

____

____

____

____

Describe your greatest fears about turning your life over to your
Higher Power.

____

____

____

____

____

____

Now that you have turned your will and your life over to your
Higher Power, describe what you feel about this. You may consider
gratitude and listing the things for which you are grateful. You may
consider hope and the expectations that give you hope. Regardless
of these suggestions, describe what you feel.

____

____

____

____

____

____

YOUR UNDERSTANDING OF YOUR HIGHER POWER

Your task here requires you to write a response to each of the statements, below. As you consider each statement and your response to it, write responses that are honest, real, and personally meaningful to you. Just to confirm what you know already, this is about your life—and saving it. So, make this exercise an important one for you.

1. STATEMENT: I thank God for having faith in me until I can have faith in myself.

____

____

____

____

____

____

____

____

____

____

2. STATEMENT: When you are in fear, you are not in faith.

3. STATEMENT: "Spirituality really is a deep sense of belonging
to life, of finding it meaningful on every level." *-Joan Borysenko*

____

____

____

____

____

____

____

____

____

____

____

____

4. STATEMENT: Humility is not thinking less of yourself, but thinking of yourself less.

5. STATEMENT: Life is God's gift to you. What you do with it is your gift to God.

____

____

____

____

____

____

____

____

____

____

____

____

6. STATEMENT: I'm sick, but I believe that God can fix what God has made.

7. STATEMENT: Let go and let God.

8. STATEMENT: Don't let the limits of your imagination stop you from seeing what God can do for you.

9. STATEMENT: The healthy, the strong individual, is the one who asks for help when he needs it.

The healthy, the strong individual, is the one who asks for help when he needs it, whether he has an abscess on his knee or in his soul.
Rona Barrett

10. STATEMENT: I know God won't give me anything I can't handle.

I just wish He didn't trust me so much.
Mother Teresa

FOUR O'CLOCK
STEP FOUR:
Taking Inventory

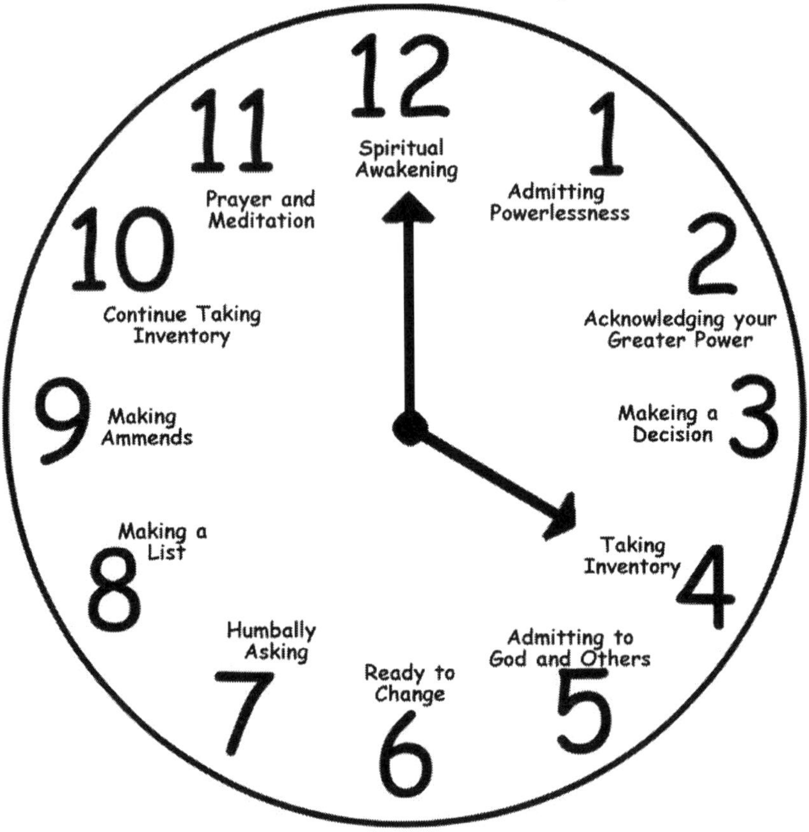

Step Four says,
"We made a searching and fearless moral inventory of
ourselves."

Step Four Prayer

Dear Lord,

The anger inside me doesn't show up much. I keep it covered, but I'm getting really tired of it. And, I have hidden sadness inside me, too. And loneliness. And shame. And defeat. And despair. And so much more that I don't want others to know about.

One step at a time hits me hard, because lately all of my steps have not gotten me anywhere that I want to go. I am afraid to take the next step.

One day at a time comes at me like a blank wall, just like all of my days, recently. I dread the next day.

One life at a time weighs pretty heavy on me, as if I have to be responsible for something that I can't manage very well.

But I have to take the next step, if I can, and I have to live one day at a time, if I can, and I have only one life to live.

And, now, I take a deep breath, knowing that I must take a necessary, serious, long, and hard look at myself, if I am going to get well and leave my addiction behind me.

So, Lord, my prayer is that you will stay with me, while I take a look at myself. When I begin to feel weak and want to stop taking a fearless inventory of myself as an addict, I ask you to give me strength.

When I feel angry and disappointed in myself, while I take a fearless inventory of myself as an addict, I ask you to give me peace.

When I feel afraid and tempted to turn away from a fearless inventory of myself as an addict, I ask you to give me courage to go on.

When I feel confused and wonder whether my life is worth living, while I take a fearless inventory of myself as an addict, I ask you to stay with me, steady my determination, and help me to believe that my life is worth living.

And, now, Lord, as I begin to take a fearless inventory of myself as an addict, I may feel lost at times, but I ask you to show me the way through it.

To get through my fearless inventory of myself as an addict, I am turning my will and my life over to you. So, my prayer is that you will stay with me. Amen.

Step Four
Lessons for You

"Why should I take a fearless inventory of myself as an addict?" If this is your question, you deserve a straight and clear answer.

In short, the answer is that recovering addicts cannot effectively manage their lives, if they are ignorant about what their lives contain. To say this in different words, some of the power of recovering addicts to manage their lives comes from knowing what there is to manage. For addicts, though, management is only part of the recovery story. At the heart of the addict's recovery is the capacity to respect one's self and to love one's self. This comes from having solid and complete information about what to respect and to love.

This sounds easier than it is. The fact is that Step Four introduces dread, anxiety, and guilt for most of those who begin it and take it seriously. After all, Step Four asks addicts to take an inventory of what they have been avoiding. They need to remember, though, that this is part of the process of gaining health.

Most addicts hide from their pain. Their selected substance has become addictive because it helps them to hide their pain, even when the substance is the most important cause of the pain.

By hiding from their pain, addicts usually develop skills in explaining their addiction to themselves. Viewed harshly, this is their way of lying to themselves. Viewed graciously, this is their way of trying to explain something that makes little sense. So, to make sense of their addiction, they point to their "difficult circumstances." Their difficult circumstances may be a "rotten relationship." It may be a job that is a burden that looks like it will go on forever.

Many addicts prefer to explain their addiction, by fooling themselves. They like to think that their addiction is not really a problem. They like to believe that they can handle their addictive substance, with no negative health consequences. They like to think that they can stop their addiction any time they want to, as if they could do this conveniently and without much effort.

Obviously, giving up these explanations is not easy. Because a searching and fearless personal inventory is difficult, many addicts want to escape from it. They make the life-and-death mistake of dropping out of their recovery. The temptation for this is understandable, just like the temptation to avoid necessary major surgery is understandable. While the temptation to drop out of recovery may be understandable, recovery is still necessity, if the addict wants to live.

Step Four, then, takes addicts through a process of gaining important personal information about themselves. Because they feel bad about themselves, they often but falsely believe that their searching and fearless inventory should require them to expose themselves in a hostile and self-blaming manner. If some hostility and self-blaming did not emerge with the inventory, this would be a surprise. After all, addicts usually have a history of poor behavior with which they are not pleased. However, a searching and fearless inventory should also expose personal needs—such as a need for affection or companionship—and personal assets and strengths. These positive aspects of the addict sometimes come as a surprise because the addict has hidden these things from himself or herself.

Addicts in recovery need to keep in mind that finding fault with themselves is easier than finding faith in themselves. Both are necessary, though.

Exposing yourself through a searching and fearless inventory need purpose. Otherwise, it is mere exposure. Best used, though, Step Four helps addicts to heal from their pain, fear, guilt, and irrational beliefs.

Because of this, Step Four is often called "the healing Step." To be the healing Step for you, you need to think of it as more a matter of heart than of mind. It is more a matter of actively participating in your healing than of gathering information about yourself. It is more a matter of deep awareness than of a high volume of information.

So, go deep within yourself. As selfish as this may appear to be, it isn't. It is a matter of healing and of making life better for you. Keep in mind that healing is good.

Keep in mind, too, that Step Four is a process that will continue for the rest of your life. Like many important parts of your life that you have begun, taking inventory, just like learning to read, will continue for the rest of your life. With practice—along with honesty, completeness, and fearlessness—taking inventory will get easier and increasingly satisfying for you.

As you practice taking inventory of yourself as an addict, you will gain skill in doing it. You will gain skill in focusing on matters that are important to you. You will gain skill in establishing useful boundaries between yourself and others, so that they do not have the ability to manipulate you into being an active addict. You will gain skill in relating with others in ways that meet your needs and that meets their needs. You will gain skill in self-management. These are just some of the skills that you will gain. Altogether, these skills raise your level of effective self-responsibility.

The searching and fearless inventory in this workbook gives attention to spiritual matters. However, your recovery should involve some other kinds of inventories. This workbook asks you to take a searching and fearless inventory about your spiritual life, but here are some other aspects of your life that should be inventoried:

- An honest history of your addiction
- An honest history the relationships that shaped your character
- An honest account of your important personal relationships
- A serious and accurate account of what you have done wrong as an addict
- A fearless statement about how others have wronged you
- A respectful and truthful report about your personal assets
- A factual and personally real picture of your difficult personal feelings and needs that are not met

With regard to these aspects of your searching and fearless personal inventory, get help from someone who can help you with them. This may be a counselor or a chaplain or another skilled professional. Also, it may be someone who has maintained his or her recovery for a considerable period of time.

Like everything else in your recovery, you need to enter this Step with an attitude of honesty and determination. You need to enter Step Four with the expectation of searching and being fearless in taking your inventory, but not of being perfect. Perfection and recovery do not go together. After all, perfection would be a pretty radical change in the life of an addict, wouldn't it.

In this workbook your searching and fearless inventory gives attention to your spiritual life. So, please proceed to the exercise, below, for your spiritual inventory.

YOUR SPIRITUAL INVENTORY

A searching and fearless spiritual inventory may not be inviting for you. However, it is necessary, as a part of your recovery from addictions. The inventory below takes you through a list of questions. The questions are not as important as your answers. The questions are easy. The answers are challenging.

Of course, some of the questions will not be challenging for you. None of them have to be challenging. This is up to you. If you wish to recover from your addiction, you will need to make them challenging. Yes, as destructive as your addiction is or can be, you will need to gather your energy and confront yourself, by calling on your determination to get your health back, your intelligence to re-gain your sanity, and your heart to reclaim your spiritual life. Your life is worth the effort, even if this is difficult for you. Recovering your health is worth the effort. So, as you read each question and give responses to them, take each one seriously, as if your life depended on it—because your life may depend on it.

Your inventory should cover many aspects of your spiritual life. It should include an inventory of your personal belief, your personal faith, your role in your religious community, your spiritual practices, and the future of your spiritual life. These are the issues that are covered in the inventory, below.

To complete this inventory, your work may be stated in a simple manner. In short, you need to respond to the questions, below. After you have responded to the questions, you will need to evaluate your responses. Please, proceed to respond to the questions.

QUESTION RESPONSE
[Circle the best one.]

Scale

Almost Always True		Sometimes True		Almost Never True
1	2	3	4	5

Spiritual healing comes from God.

1   2   3   4   5

I believe that people can have a close personal relationship with God.

1   2   3   4   5

Most persons have a spiritual life.

1   2   3   4   5

My church provides ways to help people make sense of life.

1   2   3   4   5

Addressing "unfinished business" is an important part of personal faith.

1   2   3   4   5

I believe that God likes to see us struggle.

1   2   3   4   5

I believe that God alone gives meaning to people's lives.

1   2   3   4   5

Having faith means that you earn points with God.

        1   2   3   4   5

I believe that people have fulfilled lives because of their faith in God.

        1   2   3   4   5

My church teaches me what I need to know about God and living in faith.

        1   2   3   4   5

I believe that hard work makes faith stronger.

        1   2   3   4   5

I believe that God is a loving presence

        1   2   3   4   5

I believe that God sets the rules and that I should follow them.

        1   2   3   4   5

I believe that God will fail us, if we fail God.

        1   2   3   4   5

Churches are institutions for hypocrites.

        1   2   3   4   5

I believe that God loves people just as they are.

        1   2   3   4   5

I believe that God punishes those who do wrong.

        1   2   3   4   5

My church demonstrates the grace and love that I expect of God.

1   2   3   4   5

I believe that doubt about God is normal.

1   2   3   4   5

I pray every day.

1   2   3   4   5

I frequently attend religious services.

1   2   3   4   5

I frequently read my Bible or other religious material.

1   2   3   4   5

I listen to religious programs on radio or television.

1   2   3   4   5

I feel sad because of my loss of a strong spiritual life.

1   2   3   4   5

I have been helped by people with strong faith in God.

1   2   3   4   5

God helps me to avoid temptations.

1   2   3   4   5

I feel like I am very much alone in this world.

1   2   3   4   5

I have never been close to God.

1   2   3   4   5

I feel jealous when I am around people with strong personal faith.

1   2   3   4   5

Without God, my life may have no meaning.

1   2   3   4   5

I need reconciliation with God and others.

1   2   3   4   5

I have lost all hope of a relationship with God.

1   2   3   4   5

I believe that God has treated me fairly.

1   2   3   4   5

My addiction tells me that my faith is weak.

1   2   3   4   5

God loves me, if I act in a moral way.

1   2   3   4   5

My faith helps to keep me going every day.

1   2   3   4   5

I feel like God is tired of tolerating me.

1   2   3   4   5

My doubt about God worries me.

1   2   3   4   5

Developing my spiritual life may be important, but I need to make money.

1   2   3   4   5

I am too damaged to be of interest to God.

1   2   3   4   5

I can feel the presence of God in my life.

1   2   3   4   5

I cannot please or satisfy God.

1   2   3   4   5

Without frequent prayer, I would feel lost.

1   2   3   4   5

I have a strong connection with my faith community.

1   2   3   4   5

My parents provided a strong sense of God's presence for me.

1   2   3   4   5

I have broken many promises that I have made to God.

1   2   3   4   5

I love to share time with others who have a strong personal faith.

1   2   3   4   5

I have wonderful memories from my childhood church.

1   2   3   4   5

I am angry at God.

1   2   3   4   5

I wonder how I will be remembered and who will remember me, after I'm dead.

1   2   3   4   5

I will see positive meaning restored in my life.

1   2   3   4   5

Eternal life waits for me.

1   2   3   4   5

YOUR SPIRITUAL INVENTORY, continued:

Now that you have responded to the questions, above, you have had an opportunity to think about many aspects of your spiritual life. Your next assignment is to take advantage of the work that you have done. Review your responses, above. Then, write your answers to the following questions:

1. Describe your current spiritual condition.

____

____

____

____

____

____

2. Describe your spiritual needs.

____

____

____

____

____

____

3. List your spiritual goals.

____

____

____

____

____

____

4. List the challenges, barriers, or obstacles that may interfere with your efforts toward achieving your spiritual goals.

____

____

____

____

____

____

5. Describe the role that your family will have in your recovery and in achieving your spiritual goals.

____

____

____

____

____

____

6. How will your friends play a role in your spiritual recovery?

____

____

____

____

____

____

7. Considering all that you have been through as an addict, what gives meaning to your life at this time?

____

____

____

____

____

____

8. As you pursue your spiritual goals, where may you get help and from whom?

____

____

____

____

____

____

9.List at least five of the next actions that you need to take toward your spiritual recovery.

1.____

____

____

____

2.____

____

____

____

3.____

____

____

4.____

____

____

____

5. ____

____

____

A BLESSING FOR YOU

To assist you with your spiritual recovery, here is a blessing for you:

Give yourself credit for daring to complete your spiritual inventory. You have taken an important step forward in your spiritual recovery. But there is more.

You may regain your spiritual health. When you do, praise God.
> But there is more.

You may regain a clean conscience. When you do, thank God.
> But there is more.

You may regain physical health. When you do, work for God.
> But there is more.

You may achieve emotional health. When you do, feel God.
> But there is more.

You may recover family and friends. When you do, share God.
> But there is more.

You may feel a new interest in service. When you do, serve God.
> But there is more

You may recover joy in your life. When you do, sing to God.
> But there is more.

You may feel peace of mind. When you do, live for God.
> But there is more.

You may know the wisdom of avoiding temptations. When you do, thank God.
> But there is more.

You may acquire a serene and full heart. When you do, worship God.
> But there is more.

You may find a place with the people of God. When you do, worship God.
> But there is more.

You may gain a strong sense of God's presence in your life. Have faith in God.
> But there is more.

In God, there is always more. And, you have begun to claim it.
> Bless you.

FIVE O'CLOCK
STEP FIVE
Admitting to God and Others

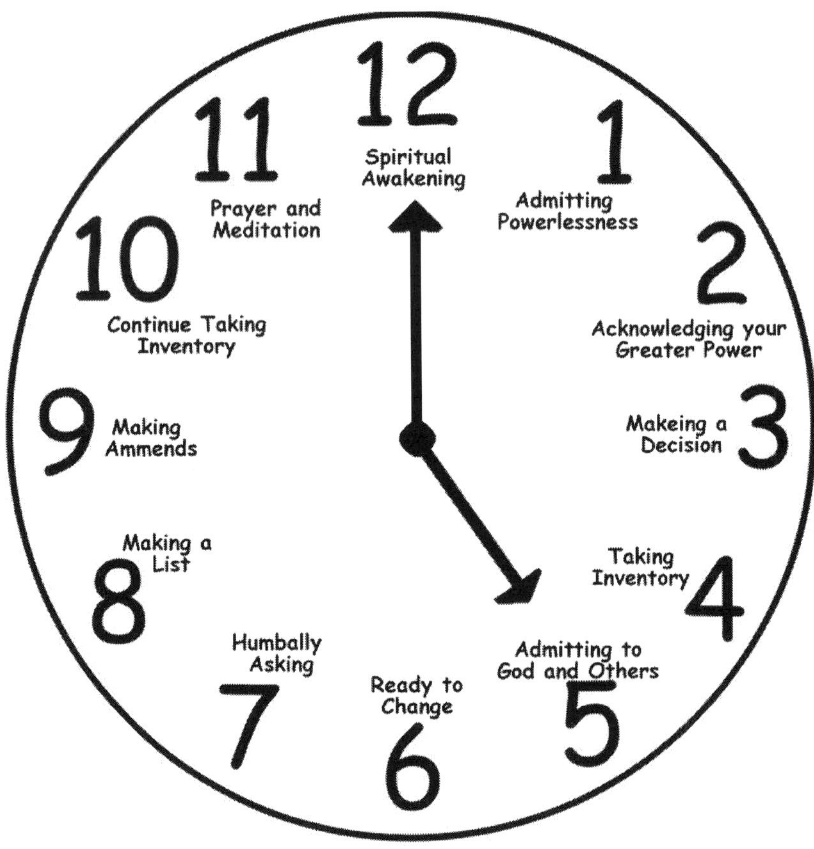

Step Five says,
"We admitted to God, to ourselves, and to another human being the exact nature of our wrongs."

Step Five Prayer

Dear Lord,

I need to admit my errors and wrongs to another person. This is difficult for me. I am not comfortable with this, but I believe that you have helped me with four out of four steps, so far, and that you will help me with step five.

So, with your help, along with my high hopes and strong determination, I will admit my errors and wrongs to another person. I have committed errors and have acted in ways that are wrong. I have done bad things. Yes, I have done bad things. And, now, I want to acknowledge my faith in you and my hope that you will see me through my recovery.

After a searching and fearless inventory of myself, I am both disappointed and encouraged by what I have found. I am disappointed because I recognize that I have hurt myself and others. I am encouraged because you have accepted me, despite my failures. I am encouraged because I hope that those whom I have hurt will accept me, too. I feel cleaner than I have felt in a long time. Thank you.

Amen.

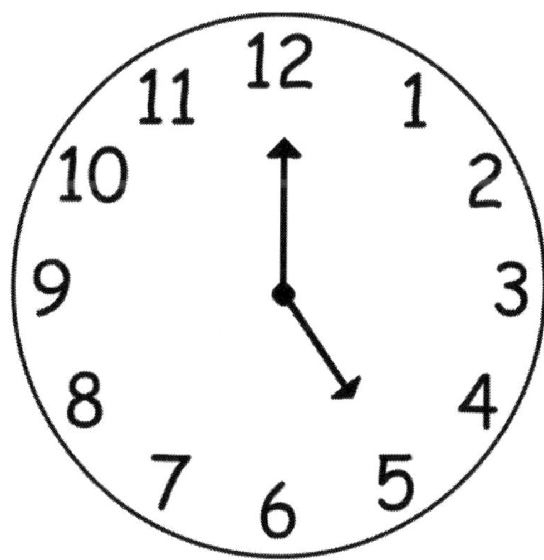

Step Five
Lesson for You

Recovery from an addiction challenges your claim to personal dignity. Step Five makes this clear. It says, "We admitted to God, to ourselves, and to another human being the exact nature of our wrongs." Despite the challenge to your claim to personal dignity, Step Five asks more of you than talking about your wrong doings. This is necessary, but Step Five is also an opportunity to reclaim your personal dignity. It is an opportunity to look another person in the eye and admit the exact nature of your wrong doings.

The lesson of Step five is a little longer than the other lessons in this workbook. It needs to be longer because it is such a crucially important step. It holds the potential of changing your life in significant ways. Just so that you may anticipate what you will learn here, Step Five is intended to take you outside yourself. If you have suffered alone with your addiction, Step Five helps you to step outside your aloneness and to begin the process of rejoining those who live in a sober world.

Step Five turns you in a new direction. After you work through the first four steps, the question is "So, what?" Does your work through the first four steps make any difference in your life? Well, maybe, not. Unless you begin to take actions to change, the first four steps will have made little difference. The difference comes in Step Five.

So, what is the new direction that comes with Step Five? In short, Step Five says that you will move outside yourself and bring another person into the process of your recovery. Actually, most of those who are in recovery have already shared their personal story with others. Usually, these include counselors, physicians, sponsors, and others who work in rehabilitation facilities and self-help groups like Alcoholics Anonymous groups.

Step Five, though, stands on the belief that "admitting the exact nature of our wrongs" will go to someone who has not heard your story.

The challenges of Step Five

Your recovery requires many changes for you. More than anything else, though, it requires you to recover from your addiction. While this step poses challenges for you, you should keep your focus on recovery. This step is another step toward recovery. So, as difficult as it may appear to be, it is necessary.

When you admit to God and others that you have harmed yourself and others, you may feel bad. And why wouldn't you feel bad? None of us wants to expose our failures. Still, feeling bad means only that you wish that you had not done things that disappoint you—a real sign that you want to be better than you have been. What would you think, if you felt great about the things you have done? The important fact to keep in mind is that just because you feel bad does not mean that you are bad. It means that you feel bad because you want to be good. It means that you feel bad because you believe in values that are better than your addiction let you be. Feeling bad is a sign that you want to be a better person.

Before you go very far into Step Five, you will want to think of the possible results of going into it.

Fear

You may be fearful as you go in to Step Five. So, you need to consider the possibility that your fears will come true. You may be humiliated. The almost never happens. Still, most individuals who seek to confess their wrong doings to another human being fear that they will be humiliated. Again, this almost never happens. Instead, those who hear your acknowledgement of wrong doing, usually respond with support and attempts to understand you and your situation.

You need to realize that this fear is normal. Neither you nor anyone else wants to expose weakness, failure, and moral lapses. Also, you need to realize that you cannot afford to let your fear get in the way of your health.

Managing your fear as a sober person may be new to you. Because of this, you need to remember that your fear can help you to be healthy, again. Yes, your fear can help you to be healthy, again.

Think of it this way: Why wouldn't you let your child play on the roof of your home? Well, the answer is obvious. You child could fall from the roof and would likely be injured, if not killed.

Your fear about what may happen to your child who plays on the roof makes good sense. Your fear helps you to keep your child safe. You keep your child from playing on the roof. Your fear tells you that you will do all that you can to keep your child safe, because you want your child to be safe. Protecting your child is more important than your fear, but the fear helps you to keep your child safe. Well, this is what your fear does for you. It keeps you safe.

If you listen to your fear, it will keep you safe. Your fear about what may happen to you when you drink alcohol again will keep you safe. Your fear of serious pain if you drive recklessly will keep you safe. Your fear of rejection by those whom you love will help you to accept them and, therefore, to be accepted by them.

But there is more. Listening only to your fear will help keep you safe, but it is not enough alone to keep you safe.

There are only two reasons to want to live. One is that you are afraid of dying. The other is that you have something to live for. So, listening to your fear is important because it will help to keep you safe. However, you need also understand that your fear tells you that you want to be safe, that you want to be healthy.

And what is the importance of being safe and healthy? Being safe and healthy allows you to listen to your needs and hopes. They will give you something to live for.

If you listen to your need for sobriety, this gives you something to live for. If you listen to your need for honest and loving relationships, this gives you something to live for. If you listen to your need for spiritual awakening and vitality, this gives you something to live for. If you listen to your need for health and feeling good about your decisions, this gives you something to live for. If you listen to your need for living a good life and sharing yours with others, this gives you something to live for.

Safety

When you listen to your fear and your needs and hopes, you're tired excuses for drinking and using no longer look good to you. Only you know what your excuses are. Some of yours may be like these:

- I drink or use because it's one of the few things I really enjoy.
- When I drink or use, I have the best times of my life.
- My drinking "friends" are the ones who matter most to me.
- No one loves me. So, why not drink or use?
- I drink or use to cover up my failures—to mask feeling bad about myself.
- It's not a problem. I can stop any time I want to. I'm always in charge.

The list of possible excuses could go on and on and on. Whatever your excuses may be, by the time you get to Step Five, they no longer help you to avoid the truth about yourself and your healthy relationships with others. So, if you no longer avoid your healthy relationships with others, what do you do? What do you do? You do something to help you to begin healthy relationships with others. You do something to re-build healthy relationships with others.

This is where you must give attention to safety.

A common assumption is that because you are sober, they will like you. They will understand that you are now healthy. Generally, this is not the way it is. You may be sober, but you do not have enough of a history of sobriety that will allow others to believe that you are healthy and welcome you into a healthy relationship with them.

You must step outside yourself. You must admit to God, to yourself, and to another human being the exact nature of your wrongs.

As you risk stepping outside yourself, keep in mind that you need to find someone with whom you are safe. Find someone who can hear your report about your wrongdoings. Find someone who can hear your struggle for recovery. To put this another way, when you admit your wrongdoings, you will likely feel deflated, as you hear yourself telling someone about truly disappointing things that you have done. This means that, as difficult as this is, you need to find someone who understands how difficult this is for you.

Keep yourself safe from yourself. When you admit your wrongdoings, you admit your wrongdoings. This means that admitting your wrongdoings does not require you to punish yourself with harsh judgments about yourself. Admitting your wrongdoings does not require you to emphasize how bad you are. Of course, you may feel bad about things you have done. This is okay and understandable. Feeling bad, though, does not make you bad. Putting yourself down with derogatory language is not necessary.

Another Person

If you are working on your Fifth Step, probably you have already discussed some of your wrong doings with others. The others have likely become trusted individuals for you. As you consider finding someone with whom you can admit "the exact nature of your wrongs," ask others to whom they have admitted their wrong doings. They can be very good sources of guidance in things like this.

Probably, you have a sponsor. Your sponsor may be your best source of advice about finding another human being with whom to admit the exact nature of your wrongs.

Many recovering addicts seek clergy for Step Five. Usually, this is a good option, for many reasons. Here are some of these reasons:

- Clergypersons have experience in receiving painful secrets from others. They are skilled in listening, but also in keeping secrets.
- Clergypersons often communicate the presence of God. They know how to speak with God and to speak on behalf of God.
- They know how to communicate grace. This means that they know how to communicate genuine care for you, even

when you believe that you do not deserve to be cared for. If you admit your wrong doings to a clergyperson, you will likely hear her/him say that you are being too hard on yourself.

- They understand human suffering better than any other profession. Because of this, they know how to handle suffering, including yours.
- They can give you spiritual language that may help you to identify some of the features of your spiritual struggles.
- They understand human weaknesses. This means that they are not going to be surprised or shocked by your confession of your weaknesses.

A Plan for Admitting

Once you have found someone to admit your wrong doings to, what do you do? How do you organize the conversation? Here are some suggestions.

- Introduce yourself, if you have not already met.
- Begin with a prayer. You may want to make some notes about what you would like to include in your prayer, but this is not necessary.
- Consider reading from the Bible. If you have selections from the Bible that are meaningful for you, consider using them at this time.
- Tell the other person what you expect from the meeting.
- Invite the other person to ask questions as you tell your story.
- Keep your story simple. Remember your fearless inventory from Step Four. Stay focused on what is important for you.
- Share honestly and openly, as if your life depended on it— because it does.
- Ask for insight, advice, and prayer from the other person.
- End with prayer.

What To Say

Remember to view the work you did in Step Four. Your fearless inventory gives you everything that you need to say to another person, when you admit your wrong doings. You may want to read your Step Four material in front of a mirror, just to get an idea about how it sounds to you and how it may sound to someone else.

In addition, here are some ideas that may be helpful.

You may want to begin your meeting with the other person by saying, "I want to confess a few things about my life that I am not too proud of!"

Here are some more ideas that you may want to use:

- "I'm looking for ways to understand what I've done and for ways to forgive myself for all that I have done wrong."
- "Generally, I have not been good at letting others help me. I need you to help me."
- "If you hear any excuses or justifications for what I have done wrong, please stop me and help me to get rid of my excuses and justifications."
- "My irresponsible drinking has caused me to hurt others. I know that I can't atone for everything today, but I would like to begin to make amends with this meeting. Help me to deal graciously with myself."

A Word about God

Step Five requires you to admit to God and another person the exact nature of your wrong doings. Like every other addict, you have found ways to avoid God. So, at this time, you may believe that God is totally absent from your life.

Maybe, the absence of God in your life is a lot like the man whose wife died. Here is what he wrote:

The Game

Underneath the guessing game
grow the thorns of doubts
that hurt when I touch
the memories of loving you.

The game.

It touches me. It leaves me
imagining forever as a peaceful retreat
from the pain of losing you.
It forges big ideas
about how pleasantly
I may be able to terminate
my torment--my grief and loneliness.
It surrounds me
with poetic pictures of bad things
that persist in causing me to wish
for a simple end to my long
and dragging depression.
It purveys the promising pause
of eternal poise, bringing an end
to the serious pain.
It invites me to join you
in your passage from this life
to something else.
It buckles my knees
from the burden of hopelessness.

And I cry.
Privately, of course.

The feeling of loss turns my head to
memories of times when I knew
your presence,
when I held you
and you held me,
when you revealed your secrets to me

and I revealed mine to you,
when we kissed,
when we talked
until we fell asleep,
remembering where the conversation
was but not remembering
who said something last.

Loss has a way of working me
into the past I shared with you.

And then I hear your voice
echoing in my head:
"Get on with your life,
you damn fool!
You ain't dead, yet."

So, one of the real messages of Step Five is this, "Get on with your life, you damn fool! You ain't dead, yet." This may be startling, but it is merely a way to say that you have a life to live, a life to give to God. Despite all wrongs that you may have done, God is still open to receiving you as a life that is worthy of grace and hope.

If you believe that you are not worthy of God's grace, this is understandable, but this does not exclude you from God's grace. It is God's option to be graceful with you, not yours.

By now, you have learned that you cannot overcome your addiction alone, all by yourself. You need others. Step Five asks you to act on this need. It asks you to be honest with yourself, with another person and with God. So, just as another person responds to you with grace and support, God will respond this way, too.

Maybe, the prayer below may help you with this:

Lord,

No one in the universe holds
as many secrets about me as you do.
     I feel safe with you most of the time,
     believing that you are love.
You take my good secrets
as well as the bad ones
and receive them as gifts,
as acts of worship.
     By hearing my secrets,
     you invite me to risk change.
When I am most honest with you,
revealing my secrets,
fearfully removing my mask,
showing you my real self,
I feel close to you, Lord,
daring to be brave, good and open,
as if I have seen and felt
your secret of eternal life.
     Even if it almost scares me to death,
     I feel like I am given life,
     a life newly conceived in eternal love,
     when I am truly honest with you.
When I am truly honest with you,
I am somehow born again.

     Amen.

Your secrets are never too bad, too awful, for God. You are never too bad for God. At this time, you are not called on to understand everything about God. Instead, you are asked to live your life. Your life needs no justification. God has already justified life. Life is good because life is good.

In addition, though, God receives your secrets, including the bad ones, as sacred expressions of life. God receives you as a sacred expression of life. This is good.

STEP FIVE EXERCISES

Write this message to yourself: "I will not expect perfection of myself." Go, ahead, write it.

____

____

____

____

Are you now willing to admit the exact nature of your wrong doings to God, to yourself, and to another human being?

______ Yes   ______ No

What did you learn from completing your fearless inventory? List five things that you learned.

1.____

____

2.____

____

3.____

____

4.____

____

5.____

As you anticipate admitting your wrong doings, what feelings best describe how you feel? Check the ones that apply to you and add others that are not listed here.

_____ guilt	_____ embarrassment	_____ fear
_____ alarm	_____ readiness	_____ jealousy
_____ resentment	_____ dread	_____ hopeful
_____ weak	_____ humble	_____ timid
_____ _________	_____ _________	_____ _________
_____ _________	_____ _________	_____ _________

Perfectionism is "stinking thinking." It is just one kind of stinking thinking, though. There are others, such as making up reasons for not admitting your wrong doings to God, to yourself, and to another human being. What are some of your stinking thoughts that could keep you from admitting your wrong doings? List them here:

____

____

____

____

____

____

____

____

Now, what is the opposite of stinking thinking? What would you say is the opposite of stinking thinking?

- Is it trying to do the right thing?
- Is it checking with your sponsor, when you are tempted to do the wrong thing?
- Is it accepting responsibility for your actions?
- Is it saying what you mean, as best you can?
- Is it honesty with yourself?
- Is it understanding that life sometimes gives you things that you cannot control?
- Is it honest regret without self-punishment?

This list of clean thinking could be much longer than it is. Now, it is your turn to make a list of clean thinking. What are some of your thoughts that are the opposite of stinking thinking? List at least ten of them.

1.____

____

____

____

____

2.____

____

____

____

3.

4.

5.

6.

7.

8.

9.

10.

Now that you have listed some of your clean thoughts, ask yourself about the advantage of clean thinking. Consider the advantages that may be involved in the positive thinking in the items, below.

Never let the fear of striking out get in your way.
George Herman ("Babe") Ruth

A pessimist sees the difficulty in every opportunity; an optimist sees the opportunity in every difficulty.
Winston Churchill

I learned that courage was not the absence of fear, but the triumph over it. The brave man is not he who does not feel afraid, but he who conquers that fear.
Nelson Mandela

Most folks are about as happy as they make up their mind to be.
Abraham Lincoln

There is little difference in people, but that little difference makes a big difference. The little difference is attitude. The big difference is whether it is positive or negative.
W. Clement Stone

The basis of optimism is sheer terror.
Oscar Wilde

That's my gift. I let that negativity roll off me like water off a duck's back. If it's not positive, I didn't hear it. If you can overcome that, fights are easy.
George Foreman

These are clean and positive thoughts. They are the opposite of stinking thinking. Consider your clean and positive thinking, when you get near to admitting your wrong doings. More than just considering clean and positive thinking, you need to ask about the advantages of clean and positive thinking. What are these advantages? Here are some of them:

- Clean and positive thinking carries the burden of hard work, but it also carries the opportunity of keeping you fresh in mind and body. Clean thinking is a lot like the way you feel after a long hot shower. You feel fresh and clean.
- Clean and positive thinking lets others know you as you are. The best evidence says that, when others know you as you are, they almost always like you. If your thinking is clean and positive, they will know you as you are.
- Clean and positive thinking lets you decide difficult issues in ways that are good for you. This kind of thinking allows you to let go of excuses for wrong doing. This kind of thinking is not merely feeling good about what you think. For example, saying "I am an alcoholic" may not feel good, but the honesty of it allows you to take better care of yourself because of your honesty about your problem. This is clean and positive thinking.
- Clean and positive thinking leads to a personal history that you can tell others about and enjoy knowing that you can tell the same thing over and over again. What a relief this is.
- Clean and positive thinking allows you to focus your energy on what is important to you. For example, instead of avoiding them or denying that they exist, this kind of thinking lets you see clean and positive people as they are and as resources for you.
- Clean and positive thinking helps you to define directions for yourself.
- Clean and positive thinking gives you the freedom with others that can lead to deep dialogue with them. The deeper and more meaningful your dialogue is, the   more likely you are to form effective connections with others.
- Clean and positive thinking allow you to be open to individuals and ideas that are stronger than yours and to learn from them. This means that clear and positive thinking can place you in situations where you are more

open to learning, more teachable, and more interested in your personal growth.

- Clean and positive thinking enables you to acquire skill in evaluating your ideas and changing them in ways that are good for you.
- In the end, clean and positive thinking equips you to make better choices.

The word of encouragement here is that your concerns about admitting your wrong doings to God, to yourself and to another human being make sense. After all, who wants to "hang out dirty laundry" for others to see? Just imagine, though, how clean and new you can feel, once you have no dreaded secrets to protect.

You know the truth about yourself. This is what you acknowledged when you did your fearless inventory. Confessing the truth about yourself makes you stronger. It sets you free from the captivity of dreaded secrets. Acknowledging the truth about yourself may be uncomfortable, but not acknowledging the truth about your self is even more uncomfortable.

Admitting the truth about yourself means that you are ready to mend your past wounds.

Now, you are ready to give yourself a new life.

Before you continue to Step Six, answer this question: What is your most important thought about your Step Five?

____

____

____

____

____

____

SIX O'CLOCK
STEP SIX
Ready to Change

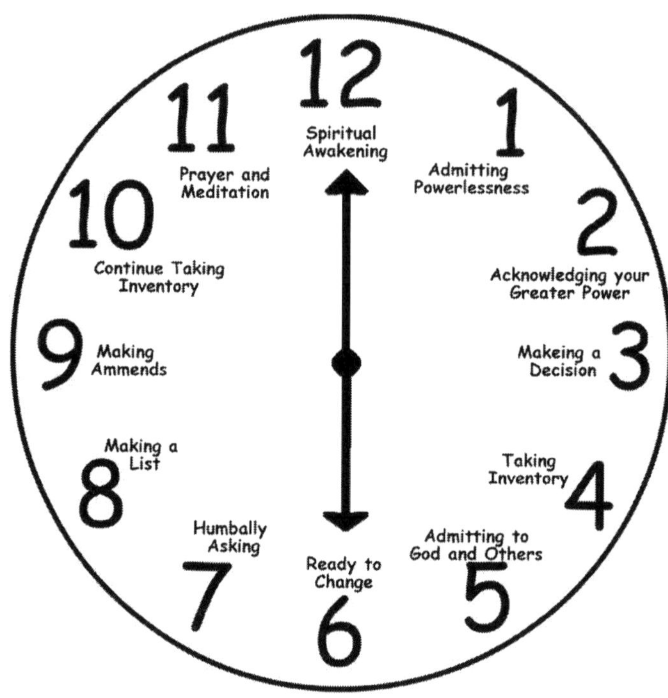

Step Six says,
"We were entirely ready to have God remove all these
defects of character."

Step Six Prayer

Dear Lord,
I am no longer willing to live with the problems that have brought me here. I ask for your help in my best effort to remove the defects of character that I now realize are an obstacle to my recovery.

I have tried to be honest with You, with myself, and with another human being. Now, I ask for your help, as I continue to honest with myself. I ask you to guide me toward mental, spiritual, and physical health.

My defects of character have stood in the way of my mental, spiritual, and physical health. Right now, my prayer is that You will stay with me, as I seek to remove all of my defects of character.
Amen.

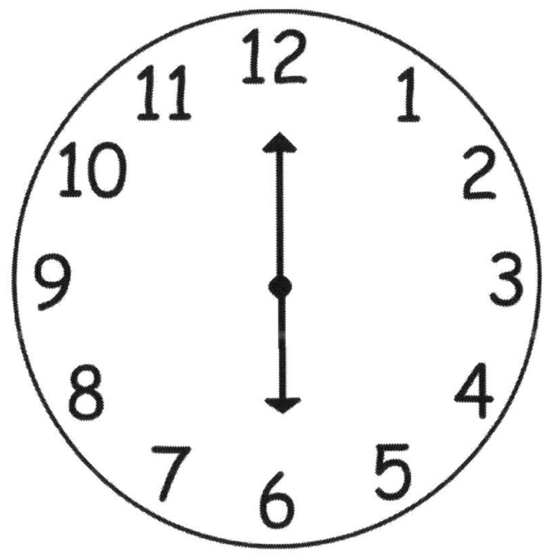

Step Six
Lessons for You

And, now, you change! And, now, you change for the better.

None of us wants to give up things that we have worked hard over a long period of time to create. This includes your defects of character.

To change, though, you need to answer two questions. One is "What is a character defect?" The other is "Are you ready to change?"

What is a defect of character? Here is the way one recovering alcoholic put it:

"Just like everybody else, I knew that I wasn't perfect. My problem was that I didn't let this knowledge interfere with trying to be perfect. So, I hid everything. I lied about everything. I got to the point that I couldn't know what I thought was true and what wasn't. I would tell somebody else whatever I wanted to, whatever I thought they would like to hear, just so they would leave me alone. And that might not have been so bad, except for the fact that I was miserable. I was a fake. I pretended at everything. And, just like a lot of other guys, I drank to keep up appearances—or so I thought. I fooled myself. I thought sometimes that I was   king of the world, because I knew that I really didn't amount to much. Nobody could love me the way I was. I was so extremely self-centered. It just never crossed my mind that I was worth nothing to anybody else. I couldn't really give anything to anyone else.

By the time I hit Step Six, I had already lost just about everything. So, I really didn't have much to give up. But, when I had to face my defects and give them up, I was scared to death. I didn't have anything else.

Now, I try not to act on my defects, but I wake up each day knowing that they are still there. And, if I'm not careful, I can drop into them again.

I did not change on my own. God opened my eyes and let me see myself. I was stunned. And now, I know that I can help others, instead of being so self-centered."

So, what is a character defect? A character defect is any personal quality that keeps you from health, love, and productive living. Here are some examples:

- Self-centeredness keeps you from taking care of others.
- Lying locks you into a stale and lifeless way of managing yourself and alienates others from you.
- Believing that you can control your drinking means that you persist in harming your body with poison.
- Living for your material comfort—even with the pain of self-abuse from drinking—prevents you from having opportunities for spiritual fulfillment.
- Dealing with others in an intolerant manner usually provokes others to become intolerant of you.

So, these examples demonstrate how certain personal qualities keep you from health, love, and productive living. Self-centeredness is a character defect that does this, along with lying, believing in your ability to control your life, materialism, and intolerance. The common and very sad outcome of practicing these character defects is that they enforce distance between you and others, between you and God.

Your attempts to remove your defects of character may frustrate you. Your attempts, though, cannot make your life worse than it is. Frustration is built in to the process of trying to change yourself.

Step Six says, "We were entirely ready to have God remove all these defects of character." Before you proceed toward having God remove all of your defects of character, go back to the Introduction to this workbook and look at the work you did on your Personal Assets. Look at the list of personal assets that you wrote. As you proceed toward dealing with your defects of character, keep your personal assets in mind.

Are you ready to change? Are you ready to have God remove your defects of character?

You are ready to have God remove your defects of character, if you can surrender each of your defects to God. This means that you recognize each of the defects as yours, that you have kept them for reasons that harm you, that letting them go may be difficult for you, and that you genuinely need to let them go. Surrender means that you accept your higher power as loving you and as ready to take your character defects from you. Surrender means that you are ready to give up your suffering and to live in a healthier manner for yourself, in a more loving manner with others, and in a seeking an open and lasting relationship with God.

More about surrender needs to be said. Your character defects may be thought of as something like acquiring a bad debt or a physical injury. You may or may not have been able to prevent it, but for now you have it. So, again, the question is whether you are ready to remove the character defects that keep you attached to your problems with drinking or drugs. Here are some additional thoughts that may help you with this:

- Your character defects may have worked for you. For example, lying to yourself about your drinking may have helped you to avoid the pain that comes with seeing that you have been hurting yourself and harming your relationships. So, surrender to change means that you accept the fact that your character defects are no longer working for you.

- When you accept the fact that maintaining your personal defects is more painful than letting them go, you are ready to surrender to a higher power.

- When you surrender to God, God removes your defects, not you. Your part is to surrender. God's part is to remove your defects. Your part is to pray and to be open to change. God's part is to remove your defects. Your part is to receive grace and support from those who want you to be healthy and loving, including God. God's part is to remove your defects. This means that you recognize that you have not managed yourself in a healthy and loving manner and that you are willing to move in the direction of letting those who are now stronger than you help you to remove your defects.

- Surrender means that you acknowledge that you are very limited. This calls for humility, based on seeing that you have not managed yourself very well. It means that you recognize how you have blocked the good will from others toward you and that you do your best to accept their good will. It means that, just as others in recovery have discovered that God can change them, you can discover that God can change you.

One of the distorted thoughts of most individuals in early stages of recovery is that they believe that once they stop drinking they are healthy. This is almost never true. The truth is that recovery is an ongoing process. It is an ongoing process that involves removing character defects, knowing that all of your defects cannot be removed all at once. This truth is based on the fact that growth and healing take time. In other words, recovery is much more a journey than a destination.

Maybe, a good thing for you to do next is to make a list of your character defects. As you do this, remember that you have personal assets and that you need to deal gently with yourself.

Probably, you already know about your character defects. Just in case you need some help in identifying them, the following list is yours to use. Here is a recommendation about how to use the list. Read each defect and rate yourself as having it or not. Then, when you are finished, make a list of those that most fit you.

DEFECT	Not Me									Me
Abrasive	1	2	3	4	5	6	7	8	9	10
Aggressive	1	2	3	4	5	6	7	8	9	10
Aloof	1	2	3	4	5	6	7	8	9	10
Angry	1	2	3	4	5	6	7	8	9	10
Apathetic	1	2	3	4	5	6	7	8	9	10
Argumentative	1	2	3	4	5	6	7	8	9	10
Arrogant	1	2	3	4	5	6	7	8	9	10
Attention Seeking	1	2	3	4	5	6	7	8	9	10
Avaricious	1	2	3	4	5	6	7	8	9	10
Bad attitude	1	2	3	4	5	6	7	8	9	10
Belligerent	1	2	3	4	5	6	7	8	9	10
Bigoted	1	2	3	4	5	6	7	8	9	10
Bitter	1	2	3	4	5	6	7	8	9	10
Blaming	1	2	3	4	5	6	7	8	9	10
Braggart	1	2	3	4	5	6	7	8	9	10
Careless	1	2	3	4	5	6	7	8	9	10
Cheating	1	2	3	4	5	6	7	8	9	10
Closed-mindedness	1	2	3	4	5	6	7	8	9	10
Cold-hearted	1	2	3	4	5	6	7	8	9	10
Compares to others	1	2	3	4	5	6	7	8	9	10
Complaining	1	2	3	4	5	6	7	8	9	10
Compulsive	1	2	3	4	5	6	7	8	9	10
Conceited	1	2	3	4	5	6	7	8	9	10
Contemptuous	1	2	3	4	5	6	7	8	9	10
Controlling	1	2	3	4	5	6	7	8	9	10

	1	2	3	4	5	6	7	8	9	10
Critical	1	2	3	4	5	6	7	8	9	10
Cruel	1	2	3	4	5	6	7	8	9	10
Deceitful	1	2	3	4	5	6	7	8	9	10
Defensive	1	2	3	4	5	6	7	8	9	10
Defiant	1	2	3	4	5	6	7	8	9	10
Denying	1	2	3	4	5	6	7	8	9	10
Detached	1	2	3	4	5	6	7	8	9	10
Dependent	1	2	3	4	5	6	7	8	9	10
Dishonest	1	2	3	4	5	6	7	8	9	10
Disorganized	1	2	3	4	5	6	7	8	9	10
Distrustful	1	2	3	4	5	6	7	8	9	10
Dominating	1	2	3	4	5	6	7	8	9	10
Embellishing	1	2	3	4	5	6	7	8	9	10
Envious	1	2	3	4	5	6	7	8	9	10
Evasive	1	2	3	4	5	6	7	8	9	10
Excessive profanity	1	2	3	4	5	6	7	8	9	10
Fake	1	2	3	4	5	6	7	8	9	10
False pride	1	2	3	4	5	6	7	8	9	10
Fear	1	2	3	4	5	6	7	8	9	10
Gluttonous	1	2	3	4	5	6	7	8	9	10
Gossipy	1	2	3	4	5	6	7	8	9	10
Grandiose	1	2	3	4	5	6	7	8	9	10
Greedy	1	2	3	4	5	6	7	8	9	10
Guilty	1	2	3	4	5	6	7	8	9	10
Hateful	1	2	3	4	5	6	7	8	9	10
Head-strong	1	2	3	4	5	6	7	8	9	10

Hostile	1	2	3	4	5	6	7	8	9	10
Humorless	1	2	3	4	5	6	7	8	9	10
Hypocritical	1	2	3	4	5	6	7	8	9	10
Immature	1	2	3	4	5	6	7	8	9	10
Impatient	1	2	3	4	5	6	7	8	9	10
Impulsive	1	2	3	4	5	6	7	8	9	10
Inconsiderate	1	2	3	4	5	6	7	8	9	10
Indecisive	1	2	3	4	5	6	7	8	9	10
Indifferent	1	2	3	4	5	6	7	8	9	10
Inferior	1	2	3	4	5	6	7	8	9	10
Insecure	1	2	3	4	5	6	7	8	9	10
Insensitive	1	2	3	4	5	6	7	8	9	10
Intolerant	1	2	3	4	5	6	7	8	9	10
Irritable	1	2	3	4	5	6	7	8	9	10
Irresponsible	1	2	3	4	5	6	7	8	9	10
Jealous	1	2	3	4	5	6	7	8	9	10
Judgmental	1	2	3	4	5	6	7	8	9	10
Know it all	1	2	3	4	5	6	7	8	9	10
Lazy	1	2	3	4	5	6	7	8	9	10
Lustful	1	2	3	4	5	6	7	8	9	10
Lying	1	2	3	4	5	6	7	8	9	10
Make up excuses	1	2	3	4	5	6	7	8	9	10
Manipulative	1	2	3	4	5	6	7	8	9	10
Materialistic	1	2	3	4	5	6	7	8	9	10
Need to be right	1	2	3	4	5	6	7	8	9	10
Negative thinking	1	2	3	4	5	6	7	8	9	10

Neglectful	1	2	3	4	5	6	7	8	9	10
Opinionated	1	2	3	4	5	6	7	8	9	10
Overly ambitious	1	2	3	4	5	6	7	8	9	10
Overly emotional	1	2	3	4	5	6	7	8	9	10
Perfectionism	1	2	3	4	5	6	7	8	9	10
Pessimistic	1	2	3	4	5	6	7	8	9	10
Petty	1	2	3	4	5	6	7	8	9	10
Possessive	1	2	3	4	5	6	7	8	9	10
Prideful	1	2	3	4	5	6	7	8	9	10
Physically abusive	1	2	3	4	5	6	7	8	9	10
Prejudiced	1	2	3	4	5	6	7	8	9	10
Procrastinate	1	2	3	4	5	6	7	8	9	10
Promiscuous	1	2	3	4	5	6	7	8	9	10
Prone to gossip	1	2	3	4	5	6	7	8	9	10
Prudish	1	2	3	4	5	6	7	8	9	10
Pushy	1	2	3	4	5	6	7	8	9	10
Quarrelsome	1	2	3	4	5	6	7	8	9	10
Rage-full	1	2	3	4	5	6	7	8	9	10
Rationalizing	1	2	3	4	5	6	7	8	9	10
Rebellious	1	2	3	4	5	6	7	8	9	10
Reckless	1	2	3	4	5	6	7	8	9	10
Regretful	1	2	3	4	5	6	7	8	9	10
Resentful	1	2	3	4	5	6	7	8	9	10
Revengeful	1	2	3	4	5	6	7	8	9	10
Rigid	1	2	3	4	5	6	7	8	9	10
Rude	1	2	3	4	5	6	7	8	9	10

Sarcastic	1	2	3	4	5	6	7	8	9	10
Secretive	1	2	3	4	5	6	7	8	9	10
Self-centered	1	2	3	4	5	6	7	8	9	10
Self-deceiving	1	2	3	4	5	6	7	8	9	10
Self-justifying	1	2	3	4	5	6	7	8	9	10
Self-loathing	1	2	3	4	5	6	7	8	9	10
Self-punishing	1	2	3	4	5	6	7	8	9	10
Self-righteous	1	2	3	4	5	6	7	8	9	10
Self-pitying	1	2	3	4	5	6	7	8	9	10
Self-serving	1	2	3	4	5	6	7	8	9	10
Selfish	1	2	3	4	5	6	7	8	9	10
Short-tempered	1	2	3	4	5	6	7	8	9	10
Slothful	1	2	3	4	5	6	7	8	9	10
Snobbish	1	2	3	4	5	6	7	8	9	10
Stealing	1	2	3	4	5	6	7	8	9	10
Stubborn	1	2	3	4	5	6	7	8	9	10
Superficial	1	2	3	4	5	6	7	8	9	10
Superior	1	2	3	4	5	6	7	8	9	10
Suspicious	1	2	3	4	5	6	7	8	9	10
Talk too much	1	2	3	4	5	6	7	8	9	10
Tardy	1	2	3	4	5	6	7	8	9	10
Thin skinned	1	2	3	4	5	6	7	8	9	10
Thoughtless	1	2	3	4	5	6	7	8	9	10
Uncooperative	1	2	3	4	5	6	7	8	9	10
Undependable	1	2	3	4	5	6	7	8	9	10
Undisciplined	1	2	3	4	5	6	7	8	9	10

Unemotional	1	2	3	4	5	6	7	8	9	10
Ungrateful	1	2	3	4	5	6	7	8	9	10
Unrealistic	1	2	3	4	5	6	7	8	9	10
Un-teachable	1	2	3	4	5	6	7	8	9	10
Unwilling	1	2	3	4	5	6	7	8	9	10
Vane	1	2	3	4	5	6	7	8	9	10
Verbally abusive	1	2	3	4	5	6	7	8	9	10
Vindictive	1	2	3	4	5	6	7	8	9	10
Withdrawn	1	2	3	4	5	6	7	8	9	10
Workaholic	1	2	3	4	5	6	7	8	9	10
Worrying	1	2	3	4	5	6	7	8	9	10
Vulgar	1	2	3	4	5	6	7	8	9	10
Vulgar Immoral Thinking	1	2	3	4	5	6	7	8	9	10

The next task for you is to gather your character defects into a list.
Use the blanks below for this purpose.

______________   ______________   ______________

______________   ______________   ______________

______________   ______________   ______________

______________   ______________   ______________

______________   ______________   ______________

______________   ______________   ______________

______________   ______________   ______________

If you need more space, just insert a sheet of paper here and continue to add to your list. Or, you may write in the margins to add to your list.

Completing a list of your character defects takes real courage. It does not feel good, but it is an act of faith—faith in yourself, in others who are helping you, and in God.

Completing a list of your character defects is a clear move away from self-centeredness and toward others and God. This is good.

Your list indicates that you are acquiring faith in your ability to change. Knowing this may make you hungry for change. Be patient with yourself, though. Your change will come, when you remain faithful to the process of change. This means that you have completed something significant with Step Six. You should rest, but not stop. You should pause to review what you have done and to share it with others.

Before you rest, though, you have one more task in Step Six. It is to pray. In the space below, write your Step Six prayer. As sources of encouragement for you, the prayers below are some that you may adopt or re-write for yourself.

Dear Lord,

Before I was born, you knew me. Throughout my life, you have known me. Beyond this life, you will know me, too, for you have made me and nurtured me for life, as a living feature of your creation.

In this moment, I ask for and expect little more than I have already received from you, for you have given me all I needed so far and have made my life better than I could have made it alone.

In this moment, because this is a challenging time for me and those around me, I come with a need for assurance that you will be with me, as you have been with me all along.

In this moment, attend to my needs and their needs, preserve us in your memory, and sustain us with your grace.

With its challenges, I am grateful for life and my relationship with you.

Amen.

____

____

____

____

____

____

Dear Lord,

As we make our journey through this life and into the next one, our prayer is that you will open our minds and hearts to love so that our homes, communities and world may be welcoming places for everyone who lives in them.

Our prayer is that you may be the Lord of Living so that what we do today matters more than looking too far ahead or too far behind and so that we find our ultimate security in you.

Our prayer is that you may be the Lord of Newness so that every day brings fresh, new opportunities for loving, challenges for growth for us, and a renewed commitment to service.

Our prayer is that you may be the Lord of Life so that our consciousness of life may prompt us to act in ways that help to sustain and enhance all life.

Our prayer is that you may be the Lord of Love so that all of us can live with an awareness of the realness of love in our lives and an ever increasing capacity to bring others into the circle of love.

Amen.

____

____

____

____

____

____

Trusting God,

You gave us our lives to live in the hand of your favor, but we call on destiny and on our self-reliance.

You gave us an earth of plenty to sustain us,

but we want more than you gave, shaming you as inadequate.

You gave us plenty for everyone, but we live as if your plenty should be reserved for some and not for others.

You gave us your love and a capacity to love, but we have persisted in manufacturing hate and war.

You gave us the ability to dream, to act as if life is a miracle, but we often choose to live dull lives, as if life may mean nothing.

You gave us more than we could ever hope for, but we often choose lives of despair.

Lord, you gave us yourself, as a sacrifice on our behalf, but we wonder whether you did enough. We choose to act on our own behalf, as if your sacrifice either was not enough or had not been made.

Lord, plant in our souls the renewed capacity to believe in the miracle of your intervention on our behalf and in each one of us as miracle.

Open our minds so that we may feel comfortable with living in the hand of your favor,

Open our wills so that we may sustain ourselves with the good work of caring for your planet.

Open our compassion so that we may provide service for those who need what we have.

Open our hearts so that your love shows in our capacity to love so that we make peace—of mind and among all persons.

Open our spirits so that we may re-discover the ability to dream and to believe in the sanctity of all life and act as if life is a miracle.

Open our future so that we can hope beyond hope from the many gifts that are more than we could have hoped for.

Open our eyes, minds, hearts, and souls to the miracle of life with which you have blessed us, again and again.

~Full Life Page 112 ~

Come, now, Lord, make us miracles, again. Renew our spirits. Fill us with consciousness of the fullness of life and the constancy of your presence.

Come, now, Lord.

Come, now, Lord, and remind us that you are here and that you never left us.

Amen.

____

____

____

____

____

____

Lord,

It rains. I get wet. I complain. Why me? And then I see the kindly eyes of my friend whose son died in Iraq. The rain doesn't seem so bad.

It gets cold. I get cold. I complain. Why me? And then I see the spirited enthusiasm of my friend who loves life. She lost her breasts because of cancer. The cold doesn't seem so bad.

I get tired. I complain. Why me? And then I remember my father-in-law whose brave and loving encounter with death showed more courage that I can imagine for myself. Tired doesn't seem so bad.

It thunders. I wake up. I grouse. Why me? And then I hear my granddaughter scream with delight when she gets new crayons. The thunder doesn't seem so bad.

I sit in slow traffic. I complain. Why me? And then I meet my friend who needs a heart transplant moving slowly but with more determination than I can comprehend. Slow traffic doesn't seem so bad.

I get bills in the mail. I worry about money. Why me? And then consider my sister who lives on a fraction of what I live on. The bills don't seem so bad.

Lord, you have blessed me. You have blessed me with rain and cold and family and friends and money and much, much more. When I contemplate all that you have given me, I wonder. Why me, Lord? Why me?

Amen.

Now, write your Step Six prayer in the space below.

SEVEN O'CLOCK
STEP SEVEN
Humbly Asking God

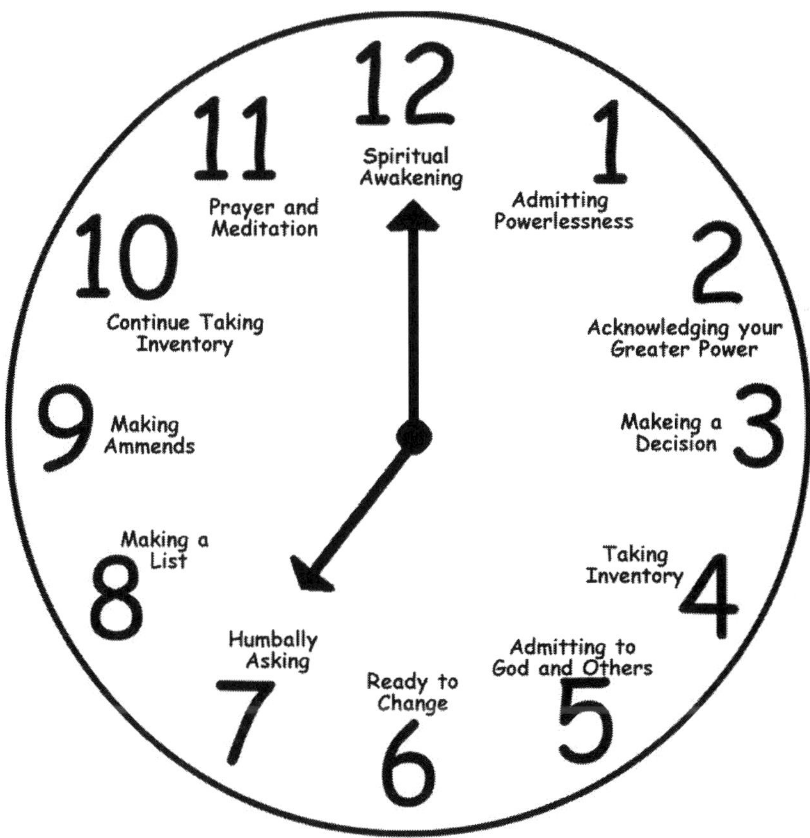

Step Seven says,
"We humbly asked God to remove our shortcomings."

Step Seven Prayer

Dear Lord,

I have hurt others and myself. Because of this, I need forgiveness. To get forgiveness, I understand that have to acknowledge what I have done wrong and to ask for forgiveness.

So, here I am. I have little to offer. I have an open mind and an open heart. Right now, in this moment, I offer them to you. I am now willing for you to take my life and manage it. I ask you to remove every defect of character. I ask you to take any skill or gift that I may have and use them for everybody's good, including mine.

I will depend on your grace and your leadership. So, as I move through Step Seven, please be with me and help me to move through it in health and love.

I will depend on others who have learned to live in a healthy and loving way. They have gone through Step Seven before me and have gained experience that I desperately need. Lord, help me to depend on them.

Lord, even if they are not deserved, for every blessing that I may receive from you, I thank you.

     Amen.

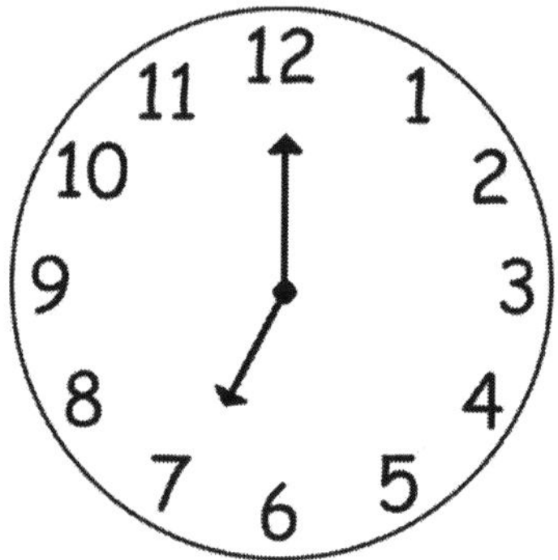

Step Seven:
Lessons for You

Step Seven calls on you to humbly ask God to remove your shortcomings. To do this, you need to ask humbly, but also to be humble. To do this, you need to be ready to let go of your shortcomings. To be ready to let go of your shortcomings, you need to be humble.

So, what does being humble mean? And, why is it necessary to be humble?

Pride, the opposite of humility, has fueled your addiction. Pride, along with self-indulgence, self-service, and many related character defects, have caused you to devote your energy to satisfying your addictive cravings. Your need for health and love was shoved out of the way by your pride.

The advantages of being humble includes the following ones:

- Being humble helps to keep you sober and clean. Following your pride cannot do this for you.

- Being humble allows you to ask your Higher Power for what you need, because you recognize your limitations in getting what you need for yourself. It allows you to appreciate God's power to transform you life.

- Being humble gives you the freedom to grow in positive ways. It helps you to break the bonds of character defects.

- Being humble provides you with the openness to receive support from others. So far, your willpower alone has not kept you sober. Receiving support from others empowers you to move toward ongoing sobriety.

If you have moved to Step Seven, humility is not new to you. Do you remember what you did in Step One? In Step One, you admitted that you were powerless over your drinking or addiction. This required humility.

Do you remember what you did in Step Three? In Step Three, you turned you will and life over to the care of God as you understand God. This required humility.

As you consider the other steps through which you have struggled, you probably recognize that you have needed to be increasingly humble. In fact, this is true, especially when you completed your fearless inventory and when you admitted your character defects to God, to yourself, and to another human being.

The point of this is that humility or being humble is a demonstration of considerable personal strength. You may feel weak in being humble, but being humble demonstrates great strength. So, now, you need to draw on your strength.

As acts of humility and strength, complete the questions below. Write what you most honestly believe and feel. This is for you. Take advantage of it.

Exercises for Step Seven

Write your personal definition of humility.

____

____

____

____

____

____

How have you demonstrated your humility?

____

____

____

____

____

____

How has your humility changed what you think and feel toward
God?

____

____

____

____

____

____

____

Describe that ways that you may be tempted to resume acting out of your character defects, such as pride, self-centeredness, lying, or others that fit you?

____

____

____

____

____

____

____

What difference does Step Seven make to you? How does Step Seven change you?

____

____

____

____

____

Humbly Ask God to Remove Your Shortcomings

This is a sensitive time. You are called upon now to humbly ask God to remove your shortcomings. To do this, here are some things that you may want to keep in mind.

Humbly asking God to remove your shortcomings is a significant sign of progress for you.

To humbly ask God for anything, especially to remove your shortcomings, reveals your vulnerability to a Power outside yourself. For most of those who do Step Seven, this is a good thing. It means that they can begin to get comfortable with their ongoing recovery. It also means that you can let go of being guarded and tense. This is good.

As you humbly ask God to remove your shortcomings, you may be feeling compassion for yourself for the first time—or the first time in many years. This alone can be life-changing.

As you humbly ask God to remove your shortcomings, you are joining a large number of men and women who now share your commitment to God and to their personal health. Remember, they feel the same insecurities that you feel, but also the same hope for the future.

How do you humbly ask God to remove your shortcomings? The short answer is this: You humbly ask God to remove your shortcomings in a way that works for you.

For you, humbly asking God to remove your shortcomings may mean only that you write one of your shortcomings on a piece of paper and toss the paper in a fireplace or in a commode.

For you, humbly asking God to remove your shortcomings may mean that you confess your shortcomings to your sponsor or another trusted person and "let go" of your shortcomings in this way.

For you, humbly asking God to remove your shortcomings may mean that you share a time of giving your shortcomings to a trusted group of individuals who share your recovery journey with you. For some individuals, the recovery group becomes the Higher Power. If this is the way you see your Higher Power, you may want to ask the group to help to remove shortcomings from you.

For most of us in recovery, though, we pray. We talk to God. We do this because we believe that God can remove our shortcomings. This is what you need to do, now. This is your time to pray. So, in the blank below, humbly ask God to remove your shortcomings.

EIGHT O'CLOCK
STEP EIGHT:
Making a List and Amends

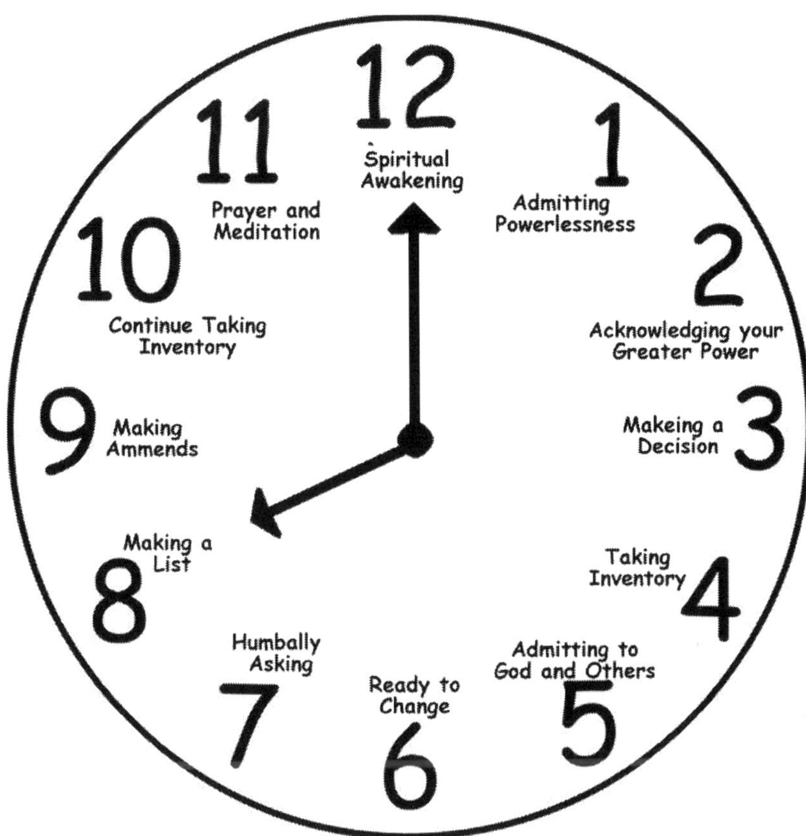

Step Eight says,
"We made a list of all persons we had harmed, and
became willing to make amends to them all."

Step Eight Prayer

Dear Lord,

I have harmed others. Right now, my concern is that I correctly list all of those I have harmed. More than making a list, though, I want to make amends so that I can help them to heal and to be healthy.

Please forgive me for the harm I have done. Please give me the courage and decency to seek forgiveness from those I have hurt and to help them to heal.

Please help me to be kind to those I have hurt and to be kind to myself as I try to make amends to them.

Lord, prepare me for any sacrifice that I may be required of me as I seek to make restitution to those I have harmed.

Thank you for every blessing, including any opportunity to make amends to those I have harmed.

Amen

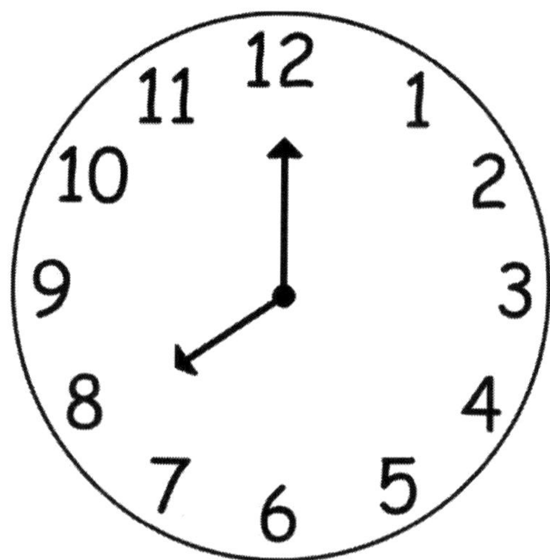

Step Eight
Lessons for You

Step Eights calls on you to make a list of all persons you have harmed and to become willing to make amends. To do this, you need to ask a couple of basic questions. One is "What is harm?" The other is "What does it mean to make amends?"

What is harm? Maybe, some questions will help you to clarify what you may mean by harm to others.

- Has anyone worried about your health and safety, because of your drinking or drug abuse? Was it you dad or your child or others?

- Have you spent money that could have provided needed benefits for others, because of your drinking or drug abuse? Were they your children or your church?

- Has anyone suffered discouragement, because of your drinking or drug abuse? Was this your spouse? Were they your co-workers?

- With whom have you been untruthful? Besides yourself, whom have you deceived? Was it your mother, your spouse, and others?

- Who needed your time and loyalty and did not get them, because of your drinking or drug abuse?

- Whose health may have been harmed because you shared drinks or drugs?

The list of questions that point to harm that you may have done could be much longer than this one.

So, what is meant by "harm?" Harm is the physical, mental, emotional or spiritual damage to other people.

What does it mean to make amends? Actually, Step Eight calls on you to become willing to make amends. The actions of making amends come later. So, for now, the question is whether you are willing to make amends. Are you?

As you add each name to your list, keep in mind that this is an important decision. As you add each name, you are moving toward a commitment to do something to make amends for the harm you have done. You are beginning to set a goal for your self.

As you add each name to your list, you are moving toward sharing your commitment with others. What does this look like to you? Is it encouraging or disturbing or disappointing or hopeful? Is it a sign of success or of failure?

As you add each name to your list, you have the opportunity of letting go of the fears that you have held inside. Once you list a name, you no longer have to hide it from your self and feel the fear that comes with the idea that someone else may know what you have done. This can be very beneficial for you.

The list that you create here is not the last one. As you continue in your recovery, you will likely remember harm that may not now come to mind.

For now, your demonstration of your willingness to make amends is that you make a list of those you have harmed.

Before you make a list of others, though, make one for yourself. How have you harmed yourself?

____

____

____

____

____

____

____

Now, make list of others you have harmed.

1. _______________________________

2. _______________________________

3. _______________________________

4. _______________________________

5. _______________________________

6. _______________________________

7. _______________________________

8. _______________________________

9. _______________________________

10. _______________________________

11. _______________________________

12. _______________________________

13. _______________________________

14. _______________________________

15. _______________________________

16. _______________________________

17. _______________________________

18. _______________________________

19. _______________________________

20. ____

21. ____

22. ____

23. ____

24. ____

25. ____

26. ____

27. ____

28. ____

29. ____

30. ____

May you continue to bless yourself with the honesty and courage that making amends demands of you.

May you demonstrate you willingness to make amends to those you have harmed so that you and they will have better lives because of you.

May you know joy and freedom from making amends.

NINE O'CLOCK
STEP NINE
Making Amends

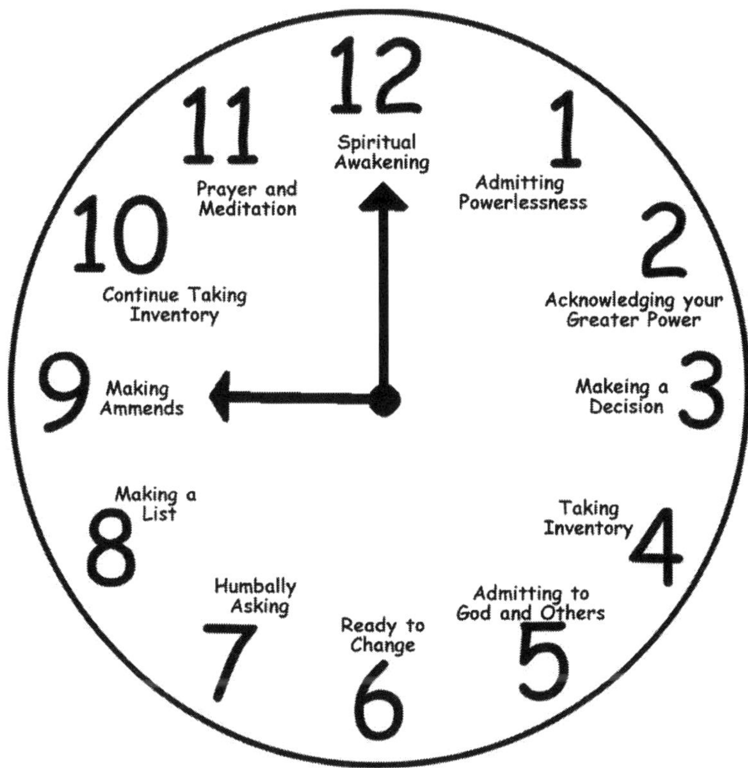

Step Nine says,
"We made direct amends to such people wherever
possible, except when to do so would injure them or
others."

Step Nine Prayer

Dear Lord,

I confess that have placed my selfish needs above others' needs, instead of helping others, and that in placing myself first I have harmed others and myself. Now, my prayer is that you will be with me and guide my thoughts and actions, as I seek to make amends to those I have harmed.

With this prayer, Lord,

> I am committing to make amends.
> I am committing to maintain my sobriety.
> I am committing to helping others.
> I am committing to actively pursue my health—mentally, emotionally, physically, socially, and spiritually.

Be with me, Lord.

> Amen

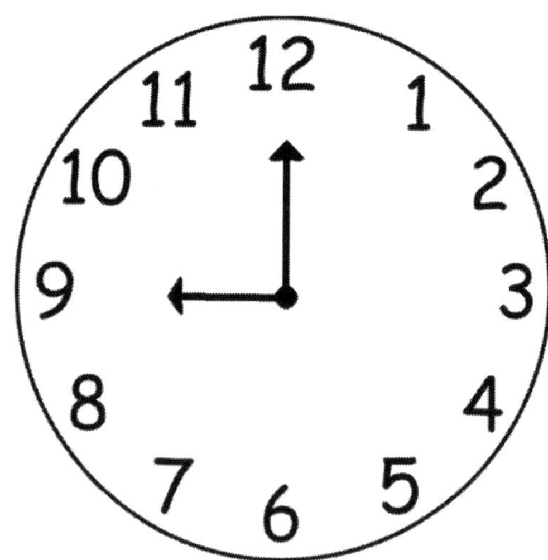

Step Nine
Lessons for You

Step Nine calls on you to make amends to those you have harmed. Generally, this means that you summon your courage, go to those you have harmed, and seek to repair the damage that you have done, except when going to them may cause additional harm.

In Step Eight, you completed a list of those you have harmed. Before proceeding with Step Nine, go the list in Step Eight. You need to do three things with the list.

First, look at each name on your list. Pray for this person. Ask for God's leadership in your consideration of making amends with this person.

Two, as you look at each name, ask yourself about what kind of damage you have done to this person. Is it mental damage, or emotional, or physical, or social, or spiritual?

Three, as you look at each name, ask yourself about whether direct contact with the person may cause more damage than you have already caused.

Go back to the list of names in Step Eight. To assist you in your decision making about whether and how to make amends, add some information to each of the names.

"M" is for mental. Place the letter "M" beside the names of individual to whom you have caused mental damage.

"E" is for emotional. Place the letter "E" beside the names of individuals to   whom you have cause emotional damage.

"P" is for physical. Place the letter "P" beside the names of individuals to whom you have caused physical damage.

"S" is for social. Place the letter "S" beside the names of individuals to whom you have caused social damage.

"S+" is for spiritual. Place the letter and the sign "S+" beside the names of individuals to whom you have caused spiritual damage.

There is more to add to your list of names. This, too, will help you in your decision making about whether and how to make amends.

Place the number "1" beside the names of individuals with whom you should seek to make amends immediately and directly. This includes individuals with whom you can "settle" things. With them, making amends is fairly complete.

Place the number "2" beside the names of individuals with whom you can make only limited or partial amends and who will need further attention than one or two contacts can give them.

Place the number "3" beside the names of individuals toward whom making amends should be deferred. These may be individuals who are hurting too much to accept any attempt to make amends. Or, they may be ones who may not be easily located. Or, they may be ones who would likely suffer more because of your contact with them than doing nothing for them.

Place the number "4" beside the names of individuals toward whom amends will never be made. Obviously, this would include individuals who are deceased. Or, they may be ones who are strangers to you.

Before doing anything else toward making amends, share your thoughts about making amends with your sponsor. Talk about each person on your list. Seek insight and advice from your sponsor and other trusted individuals who have gone before you in making amends. And, continue to pray, seeking God's direction in your recovery and in making amends.

Step Nine gives you the opportunity to right wrongs. This is a matter of sobriety, of course, but it is also a spiritual matter. It is accepting the need to get your heart right and receive the peace of mind that comes with doing the right thing. This is time to do the right thing, regardless of what the personal consequences may be for you.

Doing the right thing requires courage. The best of courage, though, runs into obstacles and frustrations. Like most of us, obstacles and frustrations provide easy reasons to procrastinate, to delay making necessary amends. Naturally, no one can give you total assurance that making amends will simply go smoothly for you. Making amends may not go smoothly for you.

Making amends, though, is not primarily for you. Making amends is for those you have harmed. Whether this goes smoothly for you or not is an important, but secondary, consideration. You are making amends for others. Therefore, you should remember that doing the right thing is its own justification—its own reward. You can guarantee whether you make amends, but you cannot guarantee whether making amends is successful.

Making amends has important benefits for you, too. Usually, those who make amends find new freedom and happiness in their lives. They do not forget their wrongdoings, but they release themselves from the burden of guilt and regret that comes with wrongdoing. Taking full responsibility for your actions is, of course, uncomfortable. However, despite the discomfort, you are likely to find a new and positive outlook on life, mainly, because in making amends you have affirmed the importance of life and living honestly and in healthy ways.

The following questions and the answers that you provide will help you to make amends in a productive, positive, and spiritually meaningful way.

What does making "direct amends" mean to you?

____

____

____

____

____

____

____

____

____

____

____

____

____

What do you expect to gain from making amends"

____

____

____

____

____

____

What is likely to be the most difficult challenge for you in making
amends to those you have harmed?

____

____

____

____

____

____

____

In what ways may prayer help you in your attempts to make
amends?

____

____

____

____

____

____

Which of your personal assets will likely enable you to make
amends successfully?

____

____

____

____

____

____

Why is making amends important to your recovery?

TEN O'CLOCK
STEP TEN
Continue Personal Inventory

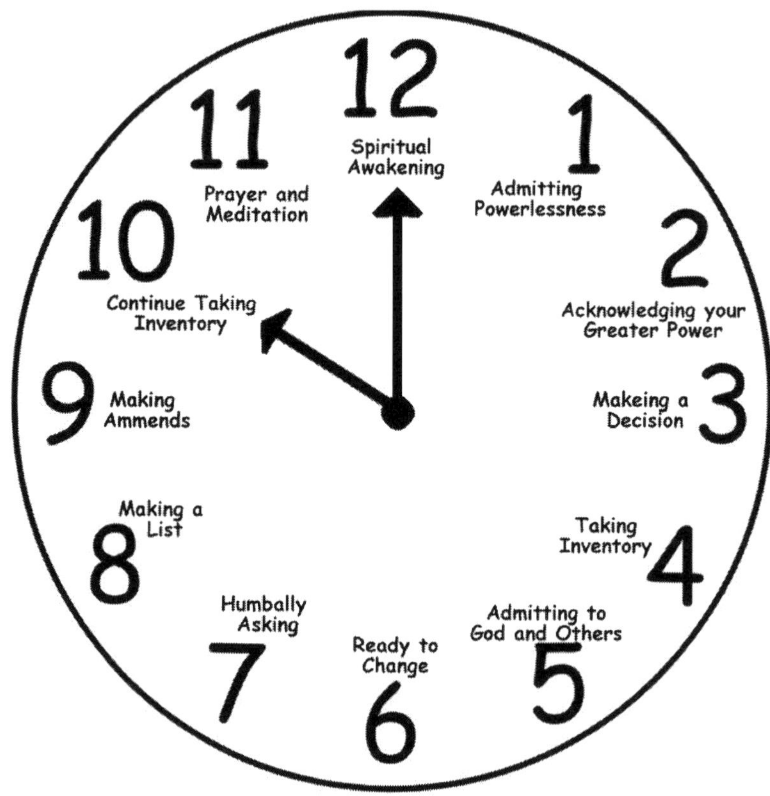

Step Ten says,
"We continued to take personal inventory and when we
were wrong promptly admitted it."

Step Ten Prayer

Dear Lord,

Today, here and now, I need your help. To continue to take a personal inventory of my character defects and my personal assets, I need your help. As I think about taking a personal inventory of my character defects and assets, I dread it because I have been working on this for a long time.

So, Lord, my prayer is that my struggle may be okay with you. I thank you for giving me a struggle that will help me to grow and to stay sober.

Lord, help me to grow in my understanding and in my willingness to change. Help me to complete my daily inventories so that my understanding and willingness can increase. Help me to see my mistakes, to promptly admit them, and to change them when I can. Help me to take responsibility for my actions, including my doubts, my negative attitudes, and wrongful behaviors.

Lord, I commit to remember to need your help and to call on you for direction that I sometimes cannot give myself. Be with me, Lord.

Amen.

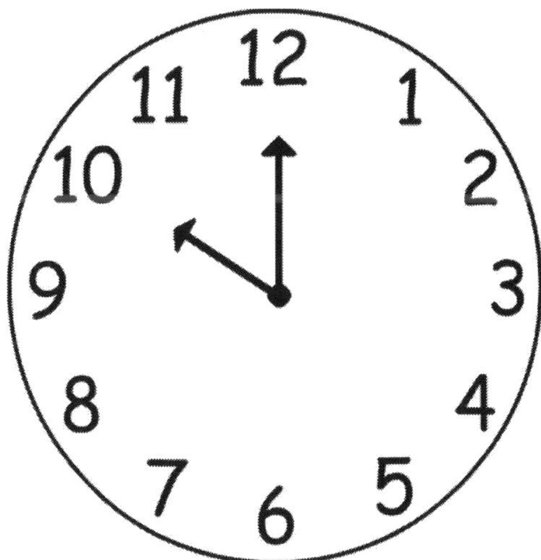

Step Ten
Lessons for You
WE

"We" includes all of us who seek health in recovery and indicates that you are now a part of us.

CONTINUED

"Continued" means that you actively participate in the ongoing journey toward health, love, and spiritual sensitivity. This is expected to last a lifetime.

TO TAKE

"To take" indicates that you willingly accept—or take—responsibility for completing your personal inventory.

PERSONAL INVENTORY

"Personal inventory" gives you a challenge. Already, you have completed a fearless personal inventory in Step Four. Mostly, your work in Step Four asked you to look back at all of the moral failures, along with ones that were ongoing at the time. Now, you are asked to pursue taking an ongoing personal inventory of your defects of character and your personal assets.

AND WHEN

"And when" tells you that at any time, you may see that you are doing wrong. Also, "and when" serves to remind you that you will make mistakes, as a matter of "when," not "if."

WE WERE WRONG

"We were wrong" calls on you to recognize that you make mistakes and that some of your mistakes are matters of doing wrong.

PROMPTLY

"Promptly" means now. At least, it means "as soon as humanly possible."

ADMITTED IT

"Admitted it" poses the opportunity to claim your health. Admitting your wrong doing to God, to yourself, and to at least one significant person, is a sign of your ongoing recovery. It is a sign of your commitment to your health and the wellbeing of others.

The outline above may make Step Ten appear to be easier than it is. Also, you have already completed a personal inventory in Step Four and you have already admitted your wrongdoings to God, to yourself, and another human being.

Step Ten requires that you move beyond what you have already done, as a way to express the growth through which you have already passed. It is re-setting of your direction so that you move in the direction of no longer fighting against your recovery or with anything or anyone else.

Specifically, Step Ten is an open door through which you enter into a new phase of your recovery that places you in a serene and less guarded frame of mind. It is knowing that you will daily take a personal inventory and that you will be ready to admit any wrongdoing. These things become your way of saying to your self and others that you have moved away from self-serving and self-centered behaviors and that, when they appear again you will promptly admit them.

Beyond taking a personal inventory and admitting your wrongdoings, Step Ten brings you to a time when you may say, "not my will but God's will be done." It allows you to endorse a style of life that is consistent with God's plan for your life. There is more to this, though.

By letting God's will set new directions for you, you will continue to move away from the self-willed behaviors that led you to self-harm and others-harm. This means that, as a part of growing your spiritual sensitivity, you will continue to ask God to remove your shortcomings and to replace them with an increasing consciousness of God's presence in your life.

In other words, taking inventory is good and admitting your wrongdoings is good, but there is more good than these. In Step Ten, you may claim some of the rewards that come with an increasing consciousness of God's presence in your life.

One of the rewards is what the *Big Book of Alcoholics Anonymous* calls "a daily reprieve." Here is the way the *Big Book* describes a daily reprieve on page 85:

"It is easy to let up on the spiritual program of action and rest on our laurels. We are headed for trouble if we do, for alcohol is a subtle foe. We are not cured of alcoholism. What we really have is **a daily reprieve** contingent on the maintenance of our spiritual condition. Every day is a day when we must carry the vision of God's will into all of our activities. 'How can I best serve Thee— Thy will (not mine) be done.' These are thoughts which must go with us constantly. We can exercise our will power along this line all we wish. It is the proper use of the will."

Another reward of God consciousness is God-consciousness itself. This is meaningful contact with your Higher Power. Here is the way the *Big Book* describes this reward on page 85:

"Much has already been said about receiving strength, inspiration, and direction from Him who has all knowledge and power. If we carefully followed directions, we have begun to sense the flow of His Spirit into us. To some extent we have become God-conscious. We have begun to develop this vital sixth sense. But we must go further and that means more action."

God consciousness increases for you as you work through Step Eleven. Just in case this seems strange to you, here is another way to think about your increasing God consciousness. It means that you have taken serious steps toward making your life better and, as a result of this, affirm life as good. The more you affirm life as good, the more you are fulfilling God's intentions for life. The more you affirm life as good, the more you are stepping into God's will.

The reference to "more action" points to Step Eleven. Before moving to Step Eleven, though, here are some tasks for Step Ten.

Step Four asked you to complete a fearless moral inventory. Step Ten asks you to complete a personal inventory. As the Big Book says, "Our next function is to grow in understanding and effectiveness. This is not an overnight matter. It should continue for our lifetime." So that you may "grow in understanding and effectiveness," here is what you need to do:

Using the chart, below, look at the last twenty-four hours. Taken from the Big Book, decide for yourself whether you have done each of the five things during each hour of the day. The five things are the following ones:

1. Continued to watch for selfishness, dishonesty, resentment, and fear

2. Asked God at once to remove them

3. You discussed them with someone immediately and make amends quickly if you harmed anyone

4. Resolutely turned your thoughts to someone you could can help

5. Showed love and tolerance of others

When you come to one o'clock, place a "Y" for Yes or an "N" for No beside one o'clock to indicate whether you did each of the five items on the list above. Place a "Y" or an "N" beside each of the five items for each hour for the last twenty-four hours.

For example, at one o'clock, did you continue to watch for selfishness, dishonesty, resentment, and fear? Beside one o'clock, put a "Y" or an "N." do this for all five items beside each of the twenty-four hours.

Go ahead.

	1	2	3	4	5
1:00	___	___	___	___	___
2:00	___	___	___	___	___
3:00	___	___	___	___	___
4:00	___	___	___	___	___
5:00	___	___	___	___	___
6:00	___	___	___	___	___
7:00	___	___	___	___	___
8:00	___	___	___	___	___
9:00	___	___	___	___	___
10:00	___	___	___	___	___
11:00	___	___	___	___	___
12:00	___	___	___	___	___
1:00	___	___	___	___	___
2:00	___	___	___	___	___
3:00	___	___	___	___	___
4:00	___	___	___	___	___
5:00	___	___	___	___	___
6:00	___	___	___	___	___
7:00	___	___	___	___	___
8:00	___	___	___	___	___
9:00	___	___	___	___	___
10:00	___	___	___	___	___
11:00	___	___	___	___	___
12:00	___	___	___	___	___

Here are some questions that will help you to reflect on the last twenty-four hours:

During the last twenty-four hours, what have you done to watch for
selfishness, dishonesty, resentment, and fear?

____

____

____

____

____

____

____

In asking God to remove your selfishness, dishonesty, resentment,
and fear, what did you say to God?

____

____

____

____

____

____

With whom did you discuss these things?

With whom did you try to make amends?

Toward whom did you resolutely turn your thoughts, for the purpose of identifying someone you could help?

____

____

____

____

____

____

____

During the last twenty-four hours, in what ways did you show love and tolerance of others?

____

____

____

____

____

____

The Lord bless you, and keep you. The Lord make his face
to shine upon you, and be gracious to you. The Lord lift up his
countenance upon you, and give you peace.

Numbers 6:24-26

ELEVEN O'CLOCK
STEP ELEVEN
Prayer and Meditation

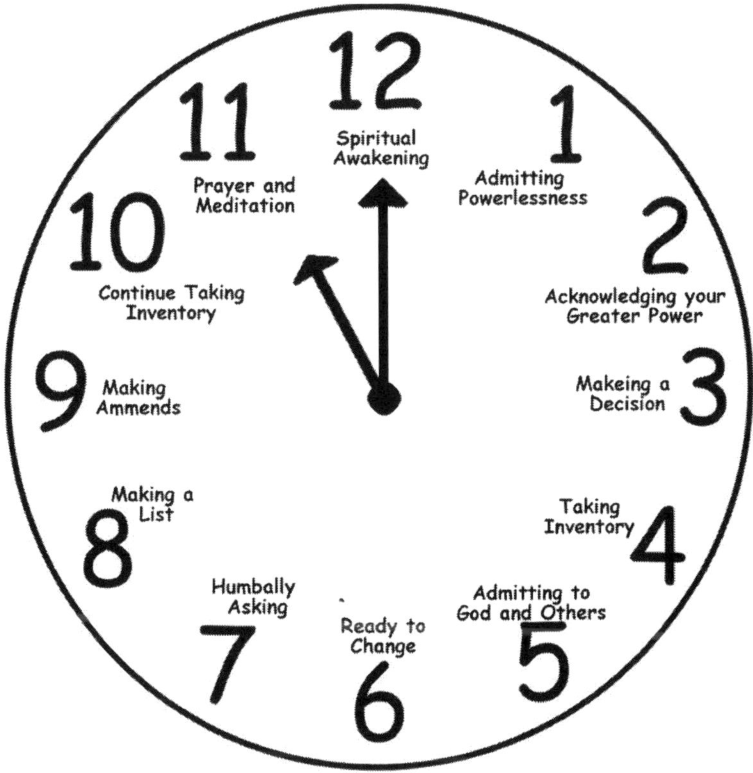

Step Eleven says,
"We Sought through prayer and meditation to improve our
conscious contact with God as we understood Him, praying only
for knowledge of His will for us and the power to carry that out."

~Full Life Page 150 ~

Step Eleven Prayer

The Prayer of Saint Francis is often referred to as "The Prayer of Step Eleven." It is provided here for you.

> Lord,
> make me an instrument of thy peace.
>
> Where there is hatred, let me sow love;
> where there is injury, pardon;
> where there is doubt, faith;
> where there is despair, hope;
> where there is darkness, light;
> and where there is sadness, joy,
>
> Divine master,
> grant that I may not so much
> seek to be consoled as to console;
> to be understood as to understand;
> to be loved as to love.
>
> For it is in giving that we receive,
> it is in forgiving that we are forgiven,
> and it is in dying
> that we are born to eternal life.
>
> St. Francis of Assisi

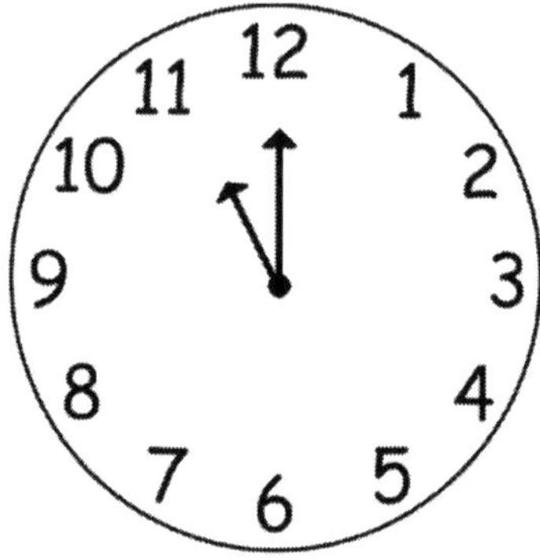

Step Eleven
Lessons for You

Here are the essential parts of Step Eleven:

> I sought through prayer
> and meditation
> to improve my conscious contact with God
> as I understood Him
> praying only for knowledge of His will for me
> and the power to carry that out.

I sought through prayer

Step Eleven confirms that you are a seeker. You seek health and wellbeing, life as God intended it for you, through prayer. To say this, though, raises the question about what prayer is. The following quotations come from The Bible, as hints about the meaning of prayer. Read each on carefully and ask what it may offer to your understanding of prayer.

> Devote yourselves to prayer, being watchful and thankful.
> Colossians 4:2

> If you, then, though you are evil, know how to give good gifts to your children, how much more will your Father in heaven give good gifts to those who ask Him!
> Matthew 7:11

> Answer me when I call to you, O my righteous God. Give me relief from my distress; be merciful to me and hear my prayer.
> Psalm 4:1

> Hear, O Lord, my righteous plea; listen to my cry. Give ear to my prayer--it does not rise from deceitful lips.
> Psalm 17:1

Call upon me in the day of trouble; I will deliver you, and you will honor me."
Psalm 50:15
The Lord is near to all who call on him, to all who call on him in truth.
Psalms 145:18

If my people, who are called by my name, will humble themselves and pray and seek my face and turn from their wicked ways, then will I hear from heaven and will forgive their sin and will heal their land.
2 Chronicles 7:14

And when you pray, do not be like the hypocrites, for they love to pray standing in the synagogues and on the street corners to be seen by men. I tell you the truth, they have received their reward in full. But when you pray, go into your room, close the door and pray to your Father, who is unseen. Then your Father, who sees what is done in secret, will reward you. And when you pray, do not keep on babbling like pagans, for they think they will be heard because of their many words. Do not be like them, for your Father knows what you need before you ask him. "This, then, is how you should pray:
"'Our Father in heaven, hallowed be   your name, your kingdom come, your will be done on earth as it is in heaven.   Give us today our daily bread. Forgive us our debts, as we also have forgiven our debtors.
Matthew 6:5-12

In the same way, the Spirit helps us in our weakness. We do not know what we ought to pray for, but the Spirit himself intercedes for us with groans that words cannot express.
Romans 8:26

Is any one of you in trouble? He should pray.
James 5:13

There are many ways to think about prayer. For those in recovery, prayer is a way to approach God with struggles for sobriety, health, and positive relationships. This means that you reveal your most intimate self to God. It means that you share your life with God, while seeking His guidance for you.

As a person in recovery, you may want to consider praying for three specific things.

One, pray for increasing and clear awareness of God's presence in your life. Two, pray for real and personal knowledge of God' will for you. Three, pray for personal strength to follow God's will for you.

And Meditation

For many centuries, meditation has been a personal discipline that spiritually sensitive individuals have practiced. Generally, meditation involves quiet contemplation. For most of us, this means that we practice being quiet, escaping the noise and clutter around us, letting ourselves feel peace, and gaining insight into matters of importance to us. For some, meditation is a quiet and relaxing experience. For others, meditation is a way to listen carefully to one's self so that hard decisions may be made. For others, it is a joyful retreat from daily pressures. For most of us, though, meditation is a quiet time during which we wait and listen for God. To do this well, we suspend our will and personal desires so that we may be receptive to God.

To Improve Our Conscious Contact with God

Like most alcoholics and addicts, when you began your recovery journey, you felt God's absence from your life, as if you had no right to His presence. Now, you have moved to Step Eleven. This is a time to welcome God's presence. It is a time to deepen your experience of God. It is a time to accept your responsibilities as a spiritual adult who pursues a consciousness of God in your life and seeks to understand His will for you.

When you began your recovery journey, you likely turned to God out of desperation. Now, you welcome God as a caring presence in your life. Now, you affirm the importance of life as good—just as God intended. Now, in actively pursuing health, the protection and improvement of life for you and others, you are fulfilling many of God's purposes for you.

To increase your consciousness of God, you will need to practice prayer and meditation. This is a life-long pursuit. Just like any other relationship, a one-time prayer or a single period of meditation is not likely to make any difference in your life. So, you will need to practice prayer and meditation so that you may build and sustain a relationship with God. God is with you. The question is whether you permit God to make himself known to you.

As We Understood Him

"As we understood Him" may suggest that God is what you understand Him to be. This is not the meaning of this phrase. If God is no more than you understand him, God is not likely to be very important.

"As you understand Him" really points to your limited understanding of God, just as the rest of us are limited in this way. We are limited in our understanding of God. Our understanding, though, is what it is. It is what we have. So, for now, we go with what we have. At the same time, we pray and meditate so that we may deepen our understanding of God. Surely, as you pray and meditate, your understanding of God will grow, your spiritual life will grow richer, and your other relationships will deepen, too. So, the phrase, "as you understand Him," is one thing now, but as you grow in your consciousness of God, will become larger and more personally meaningful.

"As you understand Him" is the beginning of ongoing change in your relationship with God. You may want to think of your understanding of God as a fertile garden that you tend with prayer and meditation. As you tend the garden, you will be reminded again and again of God's presence in your life. Over time, this will increase your consciousness of God and your fulfillment of His will for you.

Praying Only for Knowledge of His Will for Us

No one can thoroughly know God. Still, what many
thousands of men and women have discovered is that God makes
His presence known. Obviously, you have a role in discovering
God's place in your life. When you listen, God speaks. When you
obey, God acts. When you obey, God acts through you. You are
an instrument of God's will among other people. God's plan for all
of us moves forward through you and others who submit to being
instruments of life.

Among other things, this means that you submit to
discovering the good within you and letting yourself express good
to yourself and others. The good in you is much bigger than the
bad in you. This allows others to care for you, but it also allows
you to care for yourself. Step Eleven, though, short of discovering
the great good in yourself and in others, channels your attention to
a fairly simple and clear goal. The goal is that you are to pray only
for knowledge of God's will and for the power to carry it out.

And the Power to Carry That Out

In Step One, you learned that you were powerless over
alcohol or drugs. In Step Two, you accepted God as being more
powerful than you. Now, in Step Eleven, you may accept God's
empowerment of you, knowing that your strengths and weaknesses
may be ways that God uses you to demonstrate His immense
power. The important thing in Step Eleven is that you pray for
power to carry out God's will, not yours.

The Bible says, "My grace is sufficient for you, for my
power is made perfect in weakness" (2 Corinthians 12:9). The idea
that God's will may involve your weakness confuses most of us.
Maybe, this may be understood, when we consider that every one
of us came into adulthood because someone nurtured us when we
were helpless infants. Without someone to nurture us when we
were helpless infants, we would not have survived.

Maybe, another way to help us to understand power in
weakness is the example of Jesus himself. In many respects, Jesus
failed. He was prosecuted as a criminal. He was found guilty. He
was put to death. Despite these signs of failure, Jesus began a

spiritual revolution that goes on today, almost two thousand years after his death. And, those who appeared to be more powerful than Jesus—the ones who put him to death—have had no identifiable influence beyond their lifetimes. So, it is through you, including your weaknesses, that God demonstrates His power. Can you let Him do this?

Pray for power to carry out God's will. If you feel weak, consider how you may use weakness to serve God. If you feel vulnerable, consider how you may use your vulnerability to serve God. For example, is it possible that your weakness may help you to identify with and help someone else who is weak, say, because of a terminal illness? Yes, to be sure. Your weakness may help. Or, for example, is it possible that your vulnerability may help you to identify with and help someone else who is vulnerable, say, because of being unemployed? Yes, to be sure. Your vulnerability may help.

Here is a task for you, so that you may complete Step Eleven. Write your response to each of the quotations below. After you have done this, find a time when you can share your ideas with your sponsor or another trusted individual

"Don't pray when you feel like it.
Have an appointment with the Lord and keep it."
Corrie ten Boom

"Prayer is not overcoming God's reluctance,
but laying hold of His willingness."
Martin Luther.

"Those persons who know the deep peace of God, the
unfathomable peace that passes all understanding,
are always men and women of much prayer."
R. A. Torrey

"There has never been a spiritual awakening
that did not begin in prayer."

"Our prayer must not be self-centered. It must arise not only
because we feel our own need as a burden we must lay upon God,
but also because we are so bound up in love for our fellow men that
we feel their need as acutely as our own. To make intercession for
men is the most powerful and practical way in which we can
express our love for them."
John Calvin

TWELVE O'CLOCK
STEP TWELVE
Spiritual Awakening

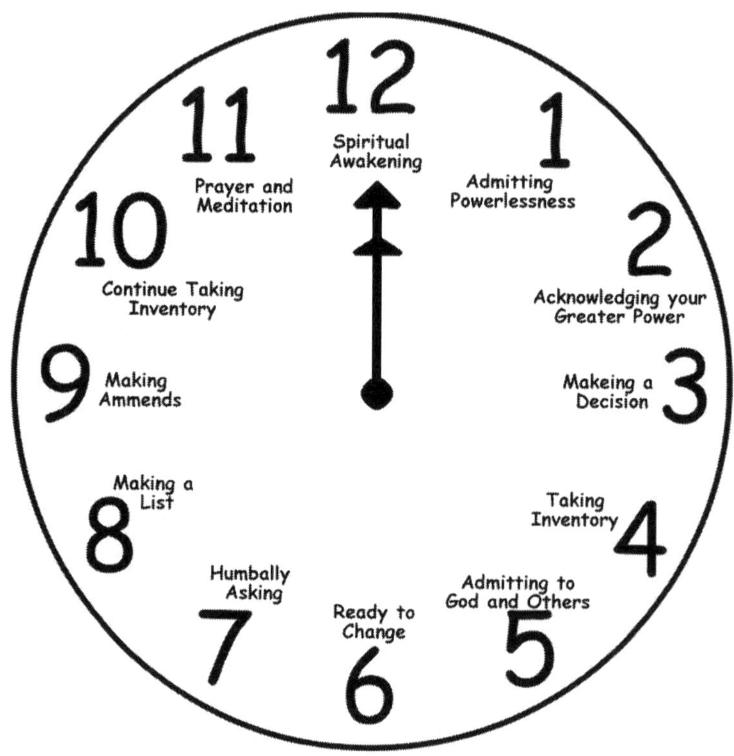

Step Twelve says,
"Having had a spiritual awakening as the result of these
steps, we tried to carry this message to others, and to
practice these principles in all our affairs."

~Full Life Page 161 ~

Step Twelve Prayer

Dear Lord,

After I said that I was powerless over alcohol/drugs, my spiritual awakening began, although I didn't know it at the time. Now, I know it. I am sober. I have a sponsor. I have friends. For all of this, I am grateful.

As my spiritual awakening continues to unfold, my prayer is that you will help me to continue to feel my gratitude and to share it with others. With your presence and power in my life, I pray for the personal determination and courage to practice the good lessons that I have learned through the twelve steps.

Lord, I need you. I need sobriety. I need friends. I need my sponsor. With all of this, I need to listen to your wisdom and theirs and to manage my behavior so that I continue my sobriety and sustain my growth toward health.

Thank you for a better way to live than I could ever have found in alcohol/drugs.

Amen

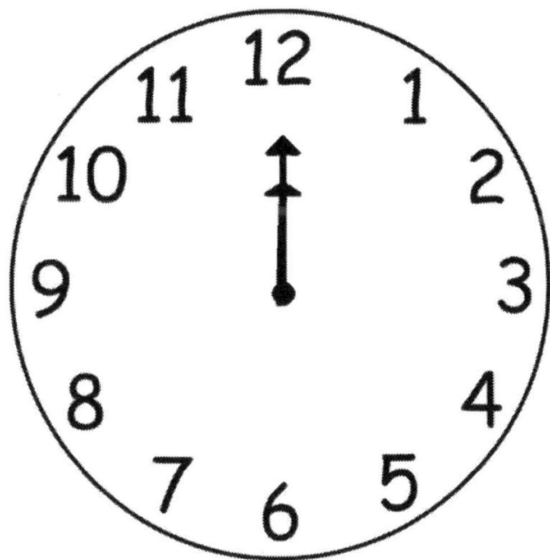

Step Twelve: Lessons for You

Your spiritual awakening began before you reached Step Twelve. How? What happened? What is this thing called "spiritual awakening?" Quite possibly, you already have the experience of a spiritual awakening, even if you don't have the words to describe what you have experienced. Here are some thoughts that may help:

Spiritual awakening may have begun when you hit bottom and recognized that the life you were living was taking you to an early death. So, instead of continuing your decline to death, you chose to live. Choosing life is a sign of spiritual awakening.

As you let others influence you, instead of trying to control everything on your own, you participated in a spiritual awakening. Letting others help you may have been the beginning of your openness to God.

Openness to a power that is greater than your power is a feature of a spiritual awakening. Your openness to God, even if you understood little about God, was likely a feature of your spiritual awakening.

When you felt deep and demanding cravings for alcohol/drugs, but didn't give in to the cravings, you experienced a spiritual awakening. Spiritual awakening requires action. Taking a stand against your cravings and for your health is real action. It says that you stand for life. Because of this, resisting your cravings empowers you.

Do you remember your first love—of someone outside your family and friends? For most individuals, some of the excitement about your first love came from the fact that someone loved you who didn't have to. Now, letting others help you with your recovery—letting them love you when they don't have to—is a sign of a spiritual awakening. Letting God love you, even when you feel like you don't deserve love, is another feature of a spiritual awakening.

Spiritual awakening is a process that flows within you. Because of this, you are the only one who can verify the truth of your awakening. If you verify it, the chances are that you have entered into a life-long process of ongoing awakening.

As you disconnect from your dependence on alcohol/drugs and establish deep connections with others, including your sponsor and new friends, you have entered into a spiritual awakening. Your connection with your sponsor and new friends is some of what enables you to connect with God.

Sooner or later, your spiritual awakening is felt and seen in your personal renewal—in your refreshed interest in life, in your concern about others and your actions toward helping them, and in your willingness to receive God in your life.

Your spiritual awakening shows in your quieting mind and heart. Instead of feeling the storm and stress of chasing after another death-inducing drink, you have stopped running. Through being quiet, your spirit is awakened.

Your spiritual awakening can be seen in your appreciation of life and in your gratitude to God for your life.

Carrying the Message to Others

Step Twelve says, "Having had a spiritual awakening as the result of these steps, we tried to carry this message to others, and to practice these principles in all our affairs." As a spiritually awake person, how do you "carry this message to others" and practice the principles of sobriety that you have learned? Providing answers to this question is your next and last task in affirming that you have entered into *Full Life*.

What is the message that you need to carry to others?

____

____

____

____

____

____

To whom do you need to carry this message?

____

____

____

____

____

____

In what ways will you carry this message to others?

____

____

____

____

____

____

____

____

Step Twelve calls on you "to practice these principles in all our affairs." What are these principles that you are expected to practice? Here is a recapitulation of these principles that you have already learned.

Early in *Full Life*, each of the twelve steps was associated with an hour of the clock. For example, Step One was associated with One O'clock. Using these associations, the principles are presented below. You are asked to indicate how you will practice these principles.

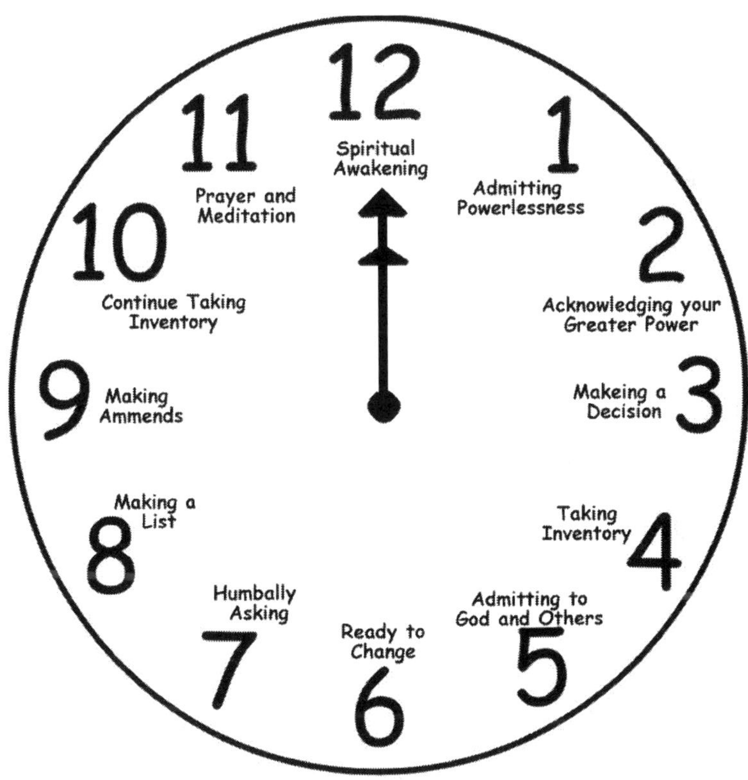

One O'clock
HONESTY

At Step One—or One O'clock—you learned that honesty required you to admit that you were powerless over alcohol or drugs. By now, your honesty has taken you several steps beyond powerlessness. The question now is this: How will you continue to practice honesty?

____

____

____

____

____

____

____

____

____

Two O'clock
FAITH

At two o'clock, you learned the principle of faith. You were invited to acknowledge your Higher Power—to express your faith in something or someone outside yourself, because of your poor self-management. The question is this: How will you continue to practice faith?

____

____

____

____

____

____

____

____

____

Three O'clock
SURRENDER

At three o'clock, you learned the principle of surrender. This means that you submitted to your Higher Power and to the belief that life is better than death. The question is this: How will you continue to practice surrender?

____

____

____

____

____

____

____

____

____

Four O'clock
SEARCHING

At four o'clock, you completed a fearless moral inventory. You practiced to search your soul and acknowledge to others what you learned. The question is this: How will you continue to practice searching?

Five O'clock
INTEGRITY

At five o'clock, you gathered your courage and admitted to God, to yourself, and to another human being, the exact nature of your wrongdoings. Representing yourself as your are is integrity. You demonstrated integrity at five o'clock. The question is this: How will you continue to practice integrity?

____

____

____

____

____

____

____

____

____

____

Six O'clock
ACCEPTANCE

At six o'clock you practiced self-acceptance, when you expressed your willingness to let go of your character defects. The question is this: How will you continue to practice acceptance?

____

____

____

____

____

____

____

____

____

____

____

Seven O'clock
HUMILITY

At seven o'clock, you humbly asked God to remove your character defects. You practiced humility. The question is this: How will you continue to practice humility?

____

____

____

____

____

____

____

____

____

____

____

____

Eight O'clock
WILLINGNESS

At eight o'clock, you expressed your willingness to make amends, by making a list of those you have harmed. The question is this: How will you continue to practice willingness?

____

____

____

____

____

____

____

____

____

____

____

Nine O'clock
FORGIVENESS

At nine o'clock, you practiced your commitment to forgiveness, by seeking it from those you harmed and giving it to yourself? The question is this: How will you continue to practice forgiveness?

____

____

____

____

____

____

____

____

____

____

____

Ten O'clock
MAINTENANCE

At ten o'clock, you committed to continue to look at your wrongdoings and character defects and to admit them promptly, as indicators of your determination to maintain your spiritual growth. The question is this: How will you continue to practice maintenance?

____

____

____

____

____

____

____

____

____

Eleven O'clock
PRAYER AND MEDITATION

At eleven o'clock, you practiced prayer and meditation, as ways to connect with God and to receive Him as you understand Him. The question is this: How will you continue to practice prayer and meditation?

____

____

____

____

____

____

____

____

____

Twelve O'clock
FULL LIFE

Now, at twelve o'clock, you have arrived at noon, mid-day—the brightest time of day. This is your bright time. It is time to feel gratitude. It is time to feel gratitude for your courage, because you faced your dependence on alcohol and your flaws. It is time to feel gratitude, because you received deep caring and support from others. It is a time to feel gratitude, because God loves you. It is time to feel gratitude, because you are affirming life as a sober person.

It is twelve o'clock. It is noon. It is bright. Life is good. Enjoy. Enjoy!

You life goes on.

Practice joy! Enjoy!

Maybe, you can claim the words of the hymn, "Joyful, Joyful, We Adore Thee."

> Joyful, joyful, we adore Thee,
> God of glory Lord of love;
> Hearts unfold like flow'rs before Thee,
> Opening to the sun above.
> Melt the clouds of sin and sadness;
> Drive the dark of doubt away;
> Giver of immortal gladness,
> Fill us with the light of day!

Now that you are at Twelve O'clock, may God fill you with the light of day!

About the Author

Francis A. Martin, Ph.D. has been in professional service as a: professor, mental health counselor, academic administrator, health care administrator, and a volunteer in mental health and medical agencies. He has written widely, with several books, including *Coping with Cancer*, *Prayers from Where You Are*, *Coping with Personal Crises*, *Vocational Guidance*, *Prayers for Recovery*, and several others. He is a frequent presenter at professional meetings, along with holding offices in professional associations. With degrees from Hannibal LaGrange College, Oklahoma Baptist University, Southern Baptist Theological Seminary, he also completed studies at the University of Missouri, University of Louisville, and Vanderbilt University.

Dr. Martin has maintained his early commitment to the effective delivery of professional mental health services. He has concentrated on his own professional development, but also on the professional development of his students, his colleagues, and members of his professional associations. In addition, he has demonstrated his long commitment to understanding and articulating a sensible, realistic, and meaningful understanding of spirituality.

6197103R0

Made in the USA
Charleston, SC
26 September 2010